A Line That Was Drawn

Copyright © 2010 Hugh Estlinbaum

ISBN 978-1-60910-245-6

All rights reserved. No part of this publication may be reproduced, stored in a retrieval system, or transmitted in any form or by any means, electronic, mechanical, recording or otherwise, without the prior written permission of the author.

Printed in the United States of America.

Booklocker.com, Inc.
2010

http://www.ALineThatWasDrawn.com

A Line That Was Drawn

Hugh Estlinbaum

This book is dedicated to those
Who supported my family
When I wasn't able to.

Introduction

When we find a soul mate to spend the rest of our days with, problems in life become easier to cope with and the good times are even more enjoyable because we have someone to share them with. That special person becomes our primary support system.

But what happens when catastrophe strikes and you're world falls apart? How much can we prepare? Sure, we can save money for downturns and missed work. We can buy that overpriced extended warranty to ease our minds. And we can spend quality time with our spouse and children in order to stay in the loop. But, where is the book telling us how to cope with our dying child?

When we first heard of the H1N1 it was something that happened to people in Mexico. By the time it made its way to the U.S., it was an underlying problem in a sea of hysteria. Being an avid watcher and reader of the media can have its down side. Drama sells. So in order to try keeping on the bright side of things, the news gets shut off, hoping a blind eye and ignorance will cure the problem.

Trying to find a balance between family, friends, work and the world is a daunting task. And then putting GOD into the mix seems to throw everything out of whack. Looking at the world we live in, with all the horrendous things happening, where is He?

He's waiting.

Chapter One

Being in a group interview at age 23 has its advantages, it's a chance to slide into a decent job and meet someone special with common goals and interests. The interview was at a restaurant called the Black Eyed Pea in the Denver area. It was for wait staff. I had worked as a cook for many years but now I wanted to try the other side of the restaurant. Not only was I successful acquiring a job, but I found a new challenge as well. Her name was Lizzy, a gorgeous auburn-haired angel, about five feet ten with a perfect figure. Graceful in all things, she was an elegant lady and the very essence of femininity. I was smitten. She was living with her Aunt Mary in Denver at the time.

Even though she was way out of my league, I thought, one doesn't get to the moon by merely ogling it. While searching for the right words to approach her, I found that every time I tried to talk to her I would stutter, and it all sounded like gibberish to me. But somehow she was able to decipher my intent. To my surprise, she said 'yes'! Sure, I was excited, but not having planned past this point, now I was distraught.

Experimenting with drugs had been my passion before meeting Lizzy. My world had consisted of bar hopping and drugs and I had never been so lonely in my life. Lizzy wasn't old enough to get into bars legally and since I was trying to find more out of life, asking her to smoke a joint or dropping some ecstasy with me made no sense at all.

Flipping through the channels I would hear people proclaiming "give it to God!" or "Jesus is the answer to all your problems!" But as for God, the closest I came to talking with Him was on the tops of 14,000 foot Colorado peaks while hiking and mountain climbing. I can say that I felt close to my creator up there. Not just by proximity, we could communicate and I could feel His spirit on those peaks. It was a spiritual thing. I would always wish the conversation lines would stay open, but reaching the bottom of the mountain was similar to hanging up the phone.

After I met Lizzy, the seedy part of my life was all over. She was my passion. All I had was my motorcycle to take her on, and the money issue of a successful date started to weigh me down. Regardless, the date ended and I felt content with my attempt. We went to a roller hockey game and then to dinner, followed by a park where we could chat. We sat in those swings enraptured with each other and prattled for hours after the sun went down; this was by far the most compelling night of my life.

Lizzy and I became exclusive and dated for about a year. She was book smart, where I was not. She was ambitious, where I was not. If it's true that opposites attract, we were living proof. I was very serious about her and I knew the future would be brighter if I had a better job. This led me to a truck driving school in Colorado. Great idea, but they wanted much more money than I had. So, I called my brother John and asked for his advice, since he was an over-the-road truck driver at the time. He said the driving schools back home in Oklahoma City would probably be cheaper. I called that school in Oklahoma City and he was right, but it was still more than I could afford. I was renting from my sister, Mandy, and brother-in-law, Tony. Tony had been my mentor, my father figure and a guiding force in my life. But now that they were selling the house to transfer to Ohio, I had to make some kind of move. That's when my brother said that if I agreed to clean up my act and go to the school in Oklahoma City, he would loan me the money.

Parting with Lizzy was emotionally draining. I had to leave the girl of my dreams, the love of my life in order to get a job that had the potential to secure a future.

The truck-driving school lasted five weeks. Not long afterwards John and I were driving over the road together, I was making good money for the first time in my life, and seeing the country. I found myself daydreaming about Lizzy. It had been about three months of driving and listening to sappy music. Jewell, the famous singer, taught me about a woman's heart and helped me realize what I had left in Colorado. I decided to call Lizzy and see how she was. It was as though we had never missed a beat. And from then on we would chat at every truck stop.

I had a load going to Cheyenne, Wyoming, and asked if she would like to meet me there. It was about a two hour-trip for her, but she loved the idea and said she would meet me there at the agreed upon time.

As I saw her walk into that truck stop, I had to take a deep breath to keep my composure. She appeared as a model with an angelic glow.

We continued to meet where we could, and occasionally I would get a load going to Denver. We were spending as much time together as we could. Her dad, Dennis, was understanding of our situation and when I would come into town he would let me stay at his house. I was growing tired of seeing Lizzy on a part-time basis, so I asked her what she thought about moving to Oklahoma City and being roommates. I think she was growing tired of the long-distance relationship too, because about a week later she said yes! I was on Cloud Nine! Having a good job and being roomies with my favorite person in the world? Life just couldn't get any better.

I called up my dad to tell him the news when he dropped a load of bricks on me. "If you want to live with her, why don't you just marry her?" he asked.

"Woahh! Hold on here, that's an awful big step!" Cold feet? I was in Oklahoma and my feet were in Antarctica! I never thought I would get married before I was forty. He said it in such a matter of fact sort of way, it got me thinking. Spending the rest of my life with this girl was in the plan, but I guess I just needed someone to talk some sense into me. My Dad has always been a source of wisdom that I admire and cherish.

After receiving her Dad's blessing, a week had passed and I was picking out a diamond ring. Another two weeks and about 10,000 miles went by with me wearing that ring on my pinky finger. I was ready to pop the question, or so I thought. I received some time off from work and asked Lizzy to meet me in Salinas, Kansas to talk about her relocating to Oklahoma. She was all for it. During the drive up there, I was filled with every emotion from confusion to anticipation. What the heck was I getting ready to do? Oh yeah! I had to get the strings needed to tie the knot! I didn't feel any better. I was shaking as though I were standing in sub-degree temperatures naked.

Lizzy and I met at a truck stop in Salinas and I can't begin to tell what the conversation was about, because my mind was way off somewhere else even though my body was there. It was as romantic of a spot as a truck stop can get. While barely able to contain myself any longer with hands shaking and blurred vision we sat at that table and I asked her to spend her life with me. For awhile the whole world disappeared, the greasy floors were no longer; the dusty curtains allowed the sunbeams to shine directly on us. Lizzy let loose a smile that drugged me like a vile of valium. I was no longer in a state of panic. It was as if I just got invited to be the honorary president of the UN. She said YES!

Seven months later we had the wedding in Denver with all our family and later we packed Lizzy up for the move to Oklahoma. My brother and sister, John and Lorie, helped with the move. John had a trailer and volunteered his help.

When we arrived in Oklahoma, I found that a week can resemble a month when it comes to waiting on a honeymoon to begin. Our first trip to Cancun, Mexico was more than we hoped it would be. We knew we were going to an "adults only" resort, but what we didn't realize was the decision Lizzy would have to make while being poolside. She opted to be unique, and leave her top on. The view (the ocean, people!) was exceptional!

After getting back to the real world we decided to go over the road trucking together and see the country. My truck was a little cramped, but being newlyweds it was more than enough room. We were traveling for three weeks when Lizzy started to get irritated at little things, and looking back this was quite bothersome, but in my opinion tolerable enough for the paycheck we would be receiving. The AC had gone out while driving through Nevada in the middle of July. It was 120 degrees outside and felt like 130 degrees inside the truck, helping us achieve a kind of slow roast-type feeling. During the time Lizzy and I were trucking over the road, we saw Maine to California. My personal favorite time was going through Southern Utah and looking to my right seeing my new bride, then looking out to see the Utah Mountains just before sunset. The vast array of colors would make me wonder how one could believe an accidental Big Bang could create something so remarkable. Thinking of that view eleven years later, I'm still in awe.

Lizzy decided to take a break from the excitement of over-the-road truck driving and wanted to set up our apartment after attending a wedding in Denver. I just looked at her and said, "Babe, whatever blows your skirt up; that's what you should do!"

After dropping her off in Denver for the wedding, I went back on the road thinking okay, maybe this isn't for us. I began to think that I needed to find something where I would be home more often. Lizzy's Dad dropped her off in Oklahoma City on his move from Denver to Tyler, Texas after the wedding.

A few weeks went by and we were living on phone calls again when Lizzy said she had some news for me. She suggested that I sit down for this one. She said, "I'm pregnant!"

It was absolutely time to come home and get a local gig. We named the little boy Tony and Lizzy made him his first shirt to come home in. It said "Made in Mexico."

Chapter Two

Before Lizzy and I were married we discussed our desire for kids, but wow - things sure can happen quickly! Tony was two years old when we decided to enlarge our family a little more, and that's when Samantha came along. Realizing the happiness these two kids were bringing into our lives, we decided to have a tiebreaker. The boys won with Zakery being born!

Being a party of five was more than what I had imagined it to be. Our times when we were all together playing games and enjoying each other were gratifying, but came with strings attached. This family of mine depended on me to bring home the bacon. Five mouths to feed required a lot of hours spent away from the house and on the clock. I thankfully found a local job that allowed me to work as much as I needed with overtime. What started out as 60 to 70 hours per week voluntary became mandatory and was expanded up to 115 hours in some weeks, when the job required it. We relied on this paycheck and I liked the men I worked with. We had a good, solid crew. My buddies and I at Dolese had many things in common; supporting our families regardless of the toll it may take on our bodies and the whole "get it done" attitude. Working for Dolese Brothers Concrete was a defining time of my life.

True, I was missing out on the time with Lizzy and the kids but at least I knew they were being taken care of with food in their bellies and a roof over their heads. Most nights with this job consisted of coming home, getting a quick bite to eat and going to bed for four or five hours so I could get up and do it again. I was happy to endure this knowing my family was taken care of and will do it again whenever needed.

It was during this time while I was working this vast array of hours that Lizzy's love and God-given patience with children led her to open a home daycare center. She called it Sunshine Daycare. It was great! She was able to raise our children while giving other children the unconditional attention they desired and needed.

When I really think about it, what is more important to a growing tree than to have a solid base and good roots? It's the same with small children. And that is what Lizzy was giving to these kids. Early childhood experience forms a base on which these kids will grow. And, wow! She did a great job, from teaching them their numbers and letters at age two and three to teaching the one-year-olds sign language so they could communicate with the world before being able to sound out the words.

Lizzy would even see a child's first steps and keep it to herself. The parents would come in the next day all excited saying they got to see their baby's first steps even though they were in daycare fifty hours a week, They got to see the first step! Lizzy wouldn't rain on their exciting day, she would just be excited with them. That's the way Lizzy was and still is.

A Line That Was Drawn

Lizzy has always been caring, patient, and puts other people's needs before her own.

There were times when she would have a colicky baby, whether it was one of ours or one attending the daycare. If it were up to me, I'd try for about fifteen minutes before my patience would run out and then I would proceed to the back bedroom, put the baby in a crib, shut the door and let them cry it out. You could say I'm not really the daycare type of guy. But Lizzy, on the other hand, would sit with that baby for hours! She would never show any impatience or frustration, but instead would just keep trying different things until something worked. Lizzy would literally love and caress the cry out of that baby. It takes a very special person to work with children on a full-time basis.

Lizzy had the daycare going for 4-1/2 when a dear friend, Felicia, called and asked for her to work at a daycare she was about to open. Seeing the opportunity to go to work and then leave it and come home is what I think enticed her into taking the job. With 2 out of 3 of our children in school now, it was a great idea. She could take the kids with her to work, the daycare bus would haul them to and from school and then come home to get personal attention from Mommy, and they didn't have to share this time with other children.

I saw all of this on a part-time basis because of the hours I was working. I was missing my family, but knew if I couldn't be there more, at least I could support them with most of their needs and wants. For awhile I was content with that, but after 3 years of the long days and nights I was enduring at work, I had to figure out how to partake in raising my children, while simultaneously keeping financially afloat.

My working buddy, Don Pratt, was in the same position. We worked the same hours and would often talk about the life we were missing out on. Don told me of a job he heard of where we could make the same money and work half the amount of time! My first thought was, "I'm not going back to the life of dodging cops again." But that wasn't the case at all; it was the real deal and I put my application in that week.

It was though I had struck gold. I was working 40 to 50 hours a week driving a truck for Sysco Foodservice and making the same, if not more, as I had been for the past three years working a sundry of hours. I was finally able to make the money we grew accustomed to and was able to have what I knew I needed in my heart; Family Time.

Chapter Three

At the present time, Tony is 10 years old. True, this story is about what our family went through during the time he was sick with the H1N1. But in order to survive all that Tony went through, strength and determination were needed; absolutely necessary. He could not have lived without it, which brings me to why Tony was so strong? Is it an accident, or maybe just good luck, as in luck of the draw type of deal? I think not.

Many may not agree with the way we raise our kids, but that's okay. My hat will come off to the one who writes a book that will explain how to raise any child. Each child is different and responds differently to disciplinary and congratulatory consequences. Lizzy and I have had many compliments on our kids' behavior. They are respectful and courteous, and they love to lend a helping hand. "Please" and "Thank you" are not foreign words to Tony, Samantha or Zakery. When going out, Tony and I often trip over each other when it's time to hold the door open for the girls in our life. All 3 of our kids have this attitude without being black and blue.

Tony was our first born, and with those who have kids, you know that the first one is the "guinea kid." We would try this or that searching for something our child would respond to. Little did we know at the time what we used with Tony wouldn't necessarily work with Samantha and Zakery; hindsight is always 20/20.

With Zakery, he definitely "challenges" us on a regular basis! Being 4 years old and the youngest of the 3 children, it's expected. He's testing the boundaries and exploring the independence he sees his siblings enjoy. Most of the time, all he needs is his shoulders redirected to the correct path. This is 99.9% of the time, but when he goes up to his momma and whacks her with the spoon and says, "I'm hungry NOW!" it's time for some Daddy intervention. Seeing this go down, I was happy to oblige. Zak needs to be reminded that it's not okay to disrespect his mother in any form, verbal or physical, so I'll tell him in a very calm voice why it's wrong to do this (remembering that he is only 4) and making sure he understands that not only do we respect others by not hitting them at inappropriate times, but we definitely don't hit women - period.

I believe using techniques like time-out for the little ones can be effective, but it's on a case-by-case basis. There are things in life that we just don't do, and at the top of that list is hitting women. Zak needs to learn at an early age while growing his roots of character the things that will not be tolerated throughout life. Warming a backside does the memory good, so with a smack on the butt he's sent to his room to think. Does he have a bruise? No! Is he a little red on his backside? Maybe pinkish. It just needs to be tacked onto his butt and know that it will make its way up to his brain. Sometimes I think his ears are there just to look cute.

With Samantha I had to learn the hard way that a whooping was not the way to get to her. Her ears are functional and adorable! There was a night when she flat out told me she wasn't going to put her dishes away after I asked her to. She was about five at the time and was there to remind me who was boss. I should have listened. I went to her and told her she needs to listen to Daddy. She just glared at me. So I picked her up by her armpits, put her over my knee, swatted her butt twice and sent her to her room. Boy, did I feel small. What the heck did I have to do that for? It's only dishes? Well, I held out for awhile, maybe 4 or 5 minutes, until I finally broke down. I went to her room to apologize for my Neanderthal behavior, but she wouldn't have a thing to do with me. I said, "Sorry baby, but what you did was wrong." She just looked at me and turned over in her bed to stare at the much more forgiving wall. I felt totally defeated; I was the bad guy that night.

That was the last time I ever thought I had to lay a hand on Samantha. From then until now in any situation all I have to do is look at her and say in a somewhat monotone voice, "Samantha, we don't do that," and she looks at me with total understanding and says, "Okay" and it's done. Thank GOD! I'd hate for her to humble me that way again.

As with many new parents with their first newborn, I was totally clueless! There was this baby looking at me as to say, "Are you going to care for me? Feed me? Love me?" Wow, if that doesn't promote you to manhood, then nothing will. And then came the "Are you going to change my stinky butt?" Uhhhh..... Lizzy, Tony needs you! Yeah, I'm a little squeamish when it comes to the downstairs plumbing! I think Lizzy is in the same ballpark as me on that one, but I've always known she's a whole lot tougher than I. As an example, I watched her go through nine months of pregnancy. The first scientist to create a womb for a man ought to be shot on sight! Watching Lizzy bearing a child with nothing? Not even an aspirin? If it were me; knock me out cold and in ten months I'll be ready to take a year off of life to recoup.

When Tony was about 2, he always wanted Mommy. I had no idea at the time why this little boy wanted to snuggle with Momma more than roughhouse with me, so I told Lizzy when he reaches the age of 4, he's going to be my boy! Lizzy looked at me, rolled her eyes and said, "Okay, whatever."

Shortly after Tony turned the big milestone of 4, I wanted to get a tattoo that said, *Ha! Told you so!* Or maybe at least a T-shirt. Fortunately, though, all that will go on my list of things thankfully not done.

Tony was just over 4 when he came up to me while I was mowing the lawn, telling me that he wanted to help. "Cool, son," I said. "Grab that bar in between the mower and me and let's get going."

He was fine with that type of work until he reached the age of 6. It was then that he looked at me and said, "Dad, I can do it myself." I pondered, and then stated, "Okay son, you can do it all by your lonesome," while turning off the lawnmower. "Start this thing up all by yourself." He looked at me a little perplexed and said, "Okay, I got it, Dad."

He pulled and pulled and pulled. After a couple of blisters he finally gave up for the day and stared at that lawnmower as if to say *"You're mine!"* He spent the rest of the summer pushing that dang middle bar with all his heart. I would keep telling him that pushing the middle bar would make him stronger and closer to his goal of starting the ornery beast. So, after every time we mowed, he would flex his muscles showing me this was his day. He started getting used to blisters from that dang pull string.

It took him until the next summer to finally start the mower. I was at work when it happened, Lizzy had been watching him and during one of his restless times, he decided to give it another go. And was he ever proud! His first major accomplishment all brought on by soul-cleansing hard work. When I came home his eyes lit up like two suns on the horizon. "I did it! I did it!" he shouted. I looked at him and told him how very proud I was that he didn't give up.

From then on throughout the rest of the summer he was able to mow the lawn by himself, always under the watchful eye of Lizzy or myself. He walked tall. It wasn't work to him; it was looking back on that lawn after finishing and having a feeling of accomplishment, not the kind you get from beating a game on the PS3, but the kind you get when you put a year of sweat and tears towards a goal.

During that same summer my father-in-law, Dennis, called and said he was coming down to see us. "What for?" I asked. "Well," he said, "to bring you some wood for your fireplace. See, I've chopped down all this wood and the lady I normally take it to here in Tyler, Texas doesn't need any more for the next two years! She's all stocked up, so I'm bringing it to you all." "Hold on here!" I said. "You're loading up a truck full of wood and driving from Tyler to Oklahoma City?" He was totally putting us before himself. That's just the type of man he is. "Cool," I said, "come on down. Tony and I will unload it when you get here."

So that weekend I see him driving up with the front wheels barely touching the ground. He had that truck loaded down way past capacity, but he didn't care. He was just happy to help out. We got him all lined up and backed into the driveway, and then the tailgate. I looked at Tony and said, "Ok let's get 'er done! I'll run and get the wheelbarrow. Get your gloves on and we'll get this knocked out in no time!"

Arriving back at the truck with the wheelbarrow, I see Dennis, but where is my son? After doing a little looking around I found him on the front porch sitting down making sure his arms still supported his head. I looked at him and said, "Hey, where's your gloves?"

"Right there, and there," he said pointing to the gloves on opposite sides of the yard, apparently put there by a good baseball arm.

"Well, go and pick 'em up, get them on and let's get to work! We don't want to be doing this in the dark."

Tony barked, "What do I care? I'm not helping you or Papa anyway!"

"Oh reeeaaally," I said, "Well why is that?"

"Because it's boring and stupid," he said.

"Man, I couldn't agree with you more, Tony, there's a chance we could drop a piece of wood on our toe. Or run over that dang cat with the wheelbarrow, not that accomplishing that would be such a bad thing."

Unsuccessfully lifting his spirits I let him know that even though it very well may be boring and stupid it's still a job that needs to be done. "And I want you to help," I told him.

"No!" he said, "I don't have to and you can't make me."

"You don't? I can't?" At this point I could feel my face getting a little flushed. My pulse rate starting to climb and my whoopin hand was ready to rock! *Man, I'm going to bend this kid over and tan his hide! One that he'll never forget! He'll wish he'd done the job like I told him to do in the first place.* With my heart racing and feeling like anything I had to say to him would be rated R, I paused for a moment. I then took a deep breath and said to him in the calmest voice I could muster "Ok, Tony, I'm not going to make you help us with unloading the wood. But, I do want you to stand by the truck and all you have to do is watch."

"Watch?" he said "Well that's stupid too!"

In my much bigger- than-me manly voice I said, "TONY, YOU ARE TO STAND OVER BY THE TRUCK RIGHT NOW!" Wondering if I was being too harsh with the boy, I got my answer; he slowly peeled himself off the front porch and as if he were fighting the much too demanding gravity, walked to the truck at a pace that I thought would make my head explode! While Tony was making sure the truck didn't turn over on its side; Dennis, Lizzy, and I worked for about an hour and a half. Zak and Samantha even challenged their muscles, seeing how big of a piece they could carry to the backyard.

After sweeping out the truck, we went to the back yard to admire our hard work and have some tea my wife had made us. While standing there talking to Dennis and Lizzy, Tony hissed, "Since everything is done I'm going inside getting me some tea and watch some TV."

"Oh no you're not, mister!"

He looked at me with a confused look on his face and said, "Well, everything's done. I'm going in now."

"No sir, you are not," I said with my much bigger than me manly voice again! "You're going to take that wood we just finished stacking and move it to the other side of the yard. And I don't mean later, right now!"

I could tell he knew I was dead serious because there were no more questions or complaints. He walked over to the wheelbarrow and while growling moved it to the woodpile.

Tony started to load it with the smallest pieces of wood he could find. I found a nice comfortable chair sat down with my sweet tea and watched. He had taken 4 or 5 loads when he ran out of the light pieces. At this time, he started to cry and was grumbling how stupid this was. He wasn't getting a response from me, however. I was drinking my sweet tea with my feet kicked up enjoying the evening.

After hauling that heavy wood for about half an hour, he looked like he was getting into the groove of things. He was not crying or pouting anymore, his movements became direct and purposeful. A couple more loads and he looked at me and said, "Look at my muscles, Dad!" I said, "Wow they are getting big! Do your muscle pose for me, Tony." Within a blink of an eye he whipped off his shirt and gave me that *Incredible Hulk* stance with all his might. Chuckling a little and admiring his newfound bulkiness, he got back to the grind of moving all that wood.

There were 2-1/2 racks of wood there for him to move but it didn't faze him a bit. He had a job and now he was determined to get it done. After 30 more minutes passed by, Tony stopped for a drink. He sat right next to me, propped his feet up and we started talking about all kinds of things other than that wood pile. With that attitude change, he became a boy who is a pleasure to be around and speak with. With our kids growing up so fast, this will be one of those times I'll look back on and smile. Not only did Tony learn about work ethics, he also had his character garden watered.

I'm learning that the older Tony gets, the fewer opportunities I'll have to shape the mold. Tony has learned that life can be hard and occasionally it can hurt, but if you put your head down and get to work you will eventually find the other side of the ditch. He popped back up and said, "Well, I'm getting back after it,

A Line That Was Drawn

Dad." It was then I knew he was good. He had a complete attitude change from a couple of hours ago. As he was walking off I hollered, "Hey, Tony, no more wood going that way. I need you to take it all back and re-stack it in the pile Papa and I had it in."

Without any questions or comments he said, "Ok, Dad!" He spent the rest of the evening moving the wood back to its original place. All while trying to form his lips to produce a successful whistle. When he was finished and I had my fill of sweet tea, we went in and sat down at the dinner table. I was looking at the boy sitting next to me; proud of him and knowing he'll make a fine man one day.

We haven't had a lot of trouble getting Tony to do work around the house since then because I think he has learned the same thing my dad taught me: Work, good sweating blister-making manual labor, does the soul good. Even now when I have something on my mind or feeling kind of blue, I find something to do, whether it's building something in my shop or grabbing the lawn mower (when Tony lets me), I'll eventually realize it'll all work out.

With Tony, I've always stressed to him to be honest, respectful and hard-working. In his early years I struggled about how to inject these values into him. I wondered what book do I need to read, what class should I take? The answer eluded me for years. I buried myself in work not knowing how to address the question. Then it dawned on me that I had already found the answer and was teaching it to the kids without even knowing it. My kids do not learn by merely telling them what to do all the time. They have to be shown. If I want them to be honest then I must be also. If I want them to be hard working then they must see me doing the same. With all the modern day conveniences we have I was really hoping to find the "Be Good Kids" button on the remote, but it's not there. Raising good, strong kids is really hard work!

Chapter Four

When Tony turned 7 in March, 2006 he started to realize that Mommy and Daddy weren't going to buy him all the stuff he wanted. He always had his needs met. Tony thought, "Dang, that new bike sure does look cool, but it's a long way till Christmas or my Birthday!" Or, "Hey, I want some ice cream off the ice cream truck! But wait, where is Mom to give me money to get it and can I make it in time?" So he took it upon himself and asked our buddy, Cody, across the street if he could mow his yard for ten bucks. Cody always took pride in his lawn and most summers it was the nicest on the block. So, it was a real surprise when Tony told me the news of his success. He wasn't all giddy and excited about the job, but said it in a real matter-of-fact going-to-get-'er-done fashion. I said, "Okay. I'll get the lawnmower filled with gas and show you how to check the oil."

I have to say, for a 7-year-old, he did an excellent job! It wasn't up to Cody's par, but watching how hard Tony worked on that lawn Cody was happy to part with the ten dollars. The next day while Tony was at school I saw Cody mowing his yard. It wasn't about the money to Cody or the loss of enjoyable work. It was about building work ethics in a generation that seems to be lacking. So many things come easy to us these days. Character will never be on that list. Tony spent that summer mowing Cody's and our lawn, making money where he could. Little did he know, people around the neighborhood saw that as a well-presented business card. The following summer he stayed plenty busy. If not mowing one of his many lawns, he was selling any service he could think of door to door.

One day, Tony and I were working on our front lawn and saw the next door neighbor's yard needing attention. I was using the weed eater and Tony was pushing the lawnmower. When trimming the fence line, I just kept on going past property lines thinking I'll just get along the fence. Well, that didn't look right so I went around the house also. I looked behind me and there was Tony not missing a beat or even having a questionable look on his face. He just kept mowing any yard I was willing to trim. We took care of four lawns that day. We didn't make any money but I believe random acts of kindness make life a little sweeter, on both ends, but especially on the giving end.

Another day Tony came up to me and said, "Dad, that lawn over there looks like crap. I asked them if I could mow it for ten dollars but he said no, he was out of work and had no money. With his lawnmower being broken, he said his father in-law was coming over this weekend and was going to mow it then. But it's Monday." Tony said, "That's almost a whole week staring at that crappy lawn."

I told him he'd just have to accept that for now and look for work somewhere else. Tony had just finished our lawn earlier in the day, so I was surprised to hear the garage door open and the lawnmower start up. After a couple of minutes I went outside to see what was going on? To my astonishment, there was Tony mowing our neighbor's lawn. "Hey, Tony, I thought the answer was no?"

A Line That Was Drawn

Tony shut down the mower came over to me and said, "I hope its okay, Dad, but right now I've got plenty of money and they don't, so I thought I'd just do this one for free. Is that okay, Dad?"

"You are one of a kind, Tony!"

With all the money Tony made that summer there sure were a lot of toys to buy. There were Games for the PS3, cool trucks, or maybe a new Nerf gun. So many decisions to be made! Well, after saving up just over two hundred dollars by late summer with only some money spent for ice cream and a few knickknacks here and there (some of them from the Boy Scout camp) I thought, "Well, I guess we'll be making a trip to the toy store soon."

Then the day came and Tony said, "I've saved up money for my new toy, Dad." I said. "Ok, son, Toys R Us or Wal-Mart? Or did you find something somewhere else?" Tony proudly said, "I did, Dad, but not at those stores. The toy I want is at Lowes. I've been doing some looking around online and found out there's a weed eater blower that's supposed to have close to hurricane power!" I had to ask, "Are you sure that's what you want to spend your hard-earned money on?"

Being 8 years old and not eyeballing an age-appropriate prize, I was thinking of taking him to the doctor to get a brain scan! He said, "I'm totally sure, Dad. If I had a blower, especially one with hurricane strength, my lawns will look like a professional's in no time!"

Since then, Tony's business has been booming! If there's something he just can't live without and he's saved up the money, then we go and get it. This surprisingly enough is pretty rare. Tony seemed to be content with life. He was very happy and anything he got into was wholehearted.

One day he said, "It's time for a new bike!" I said, "Ok, let's go." We went to the local Academy Sports and it didn't take him long to find the bike that he liked. What made it even better was that he found one in his price range; but there was a problem, when we got it off the rack we found that the chain guard had a crack in it. We told a salesman about the problem and the man immediately said, "Well that's 10% off."

"Cool!" we said unison. Ok, off to the checkout stand we go. On the way we noticed the kickstand wasn't going to work properly.

Well the salesman said, "That's another 5% off."

"Wow!" I exclaimed, "You're really going to get a deal on this one, Tony!" When we arrived at the checkout stand the cashier scanned the bar code and it rang up for $20 less than the listed price. And that's before our 15% discount! I believe that truly goes to show that what goes around comes around, for both good-hearted people and the ones who see fit to lie, cheat and steal. I believe the deal Tony received was due to his previous actions.

In our house we liked to watch football from time to time when we got a chance, and Tony had always enjoyed playing football with his buddy, Quinton, who lived behind us. While Lizzy was signing all three kids up for soccer at the YMCA, she found that this was going to be the first year they were going to implement tackle football. There was no thinking about this for Tony, even though he's loved soccer for the past three years. He stated "It's finally my time to get the game to a new level with pads and all!"

We let him know that football is an expensive sport and it will take around three hundred dollars to pay for dues and pads. I said this knowing that if Tony helps to pay for something, it will be very well taken care of and not easily lost. Without even thinking about it Tony said, "That's ok, I've got some money. Will you, Mom and Dad, split the cost with me?"

There was no second thought on this one. "Sure, son, we'll split the cost and you'll be playing in no time."

The first three weeks were devoted to hard nose conditioning. Even though he was tired from mowing lawns and going to school, he muscled his way through it with all his heart; always treating each practice as though it were the Super Bowl. Before workouts began I reminded him, "You're only going to be as good as you practice, son."

He took that to heart and gave it his all every time. Each time he made a good tackle or good block or kick he would always look in my direction and see me with a "thumbs up" or standing and cheering. I have always believed that our kids' strength and confidence rely on the support system they have backing them.

Along came the first game and boy were we stoked! Lizzy had taken Samantha and Zak to their first game of soccer. So it was my proud job to take Tony to his first football game. Our first game on September 12, 2009, was going to be a tough one. We were playing a team from Shawnee, so on the way to the game we found some good rock and roll and cranked it up. I don't know who was more excited, Tony or myself! I was slamming the air drums and Tony was rockin' the air guitar as though he was playing for an audience of 10,000 long-time fans! We were totally pumped for the first game of the season, which was for sure going to be a profound win. Well it was a blowout -- but not on our behalf. We lost the game something like 42-7. Tony was so heartbroken that he was in tears, not because of any injury, it was his first letdown after putting his all into it. A little bit of me was happy for the character he obtained, the other side of me hurt for the pain he was going through. I told Tony, "Yeah, the team lost but you came out victorious! Nobody could have asked more out of you. You gave your all and never gave up even when you tackled the kid in the end zone after his touchdown. You did great, son, win or lose you gave it your all and that's the one thing that matters to me, son." To smooth things over a little bit I said, "Let's go celebrate your personal victory at the best hamburger joint in town!"

Off to Ron's hamburgers we went. On our way there we cranked up the Rock and Roll again to continue our jam session. By the time we got to Ron's, Tony's spirits were almost back to where they were before the game! We were joined by Lizzy and the kids as well as my sister, Lorie, and my brother in-law, Mike, and had a dandy of a time talking and cutting up. All of us joined in as though it was a party just waiting to happen. Confetti was substituted with French fries and became airborne. This was the day that has changed our family's life forever...

Chapter Five

On the way home Tony started to complain of a light headache. We didn't think much about it because Tony had never been the one to get sick, maybe a cold here and there but nothing in his life that kept him down longer than a day. With a some Children's Tylenol and maybe a short nap, we thought he'd be fine. A couple of hours later he was feeling about 90%, He's always been a tough kid. Tony asked if he could invite his buddy Tommy over to spend the night. Tommy is a pleasure to be around and a well-mannered kid, so we said sure let's go get him! The boys didn't stay up too late playing games and everything seemed fine. They woke up early and started their day with a good Sunday morning breakfast.

Everything seemed normal until later that afternoon. When the headache had returned; this time it was accompanied with a barking cough and a slight fever. While I was wondering what to do for Tony, Lizzy told me that if it wasn't better by the morning she was going to get him in with our pediatrician, Dr. Crittenden, the only Doctor we've had with our children.

The next morning I went to work at my usual time, 2:30 a.m. I wasn't really worried about Tony because he was in the capable hands of Lizzy, and besides, being a father of three these things happen. Kids get sick, build their immune system, and then they get better. If I were to freak out about every cough and slight fever, I'd be a raging alcoholic by now.

With Tony feeling worse than the night before, Lizzy took him to the doctor's office. Soon after, Tony called me saying the doctor said, "I've definitely got the flu and borderline pneumonia."

He was sent home with a breathing treatment machine, which was a little odd. I mean this type of stuff doesn't happen to our kids. I thought, ok, a couple days of this and it'll be over and all will be back to normal; so I thought. After getting home, I saw Tony feeling as sick as ever! Lizzy had taken his temperature just before I walked in the door and it read 105 degrees. Knowing that's way too high, we decided to call up the on-call doctor and ask her opinion on what we should do. Not much to our surprise she said get him to the ER as soon as possible. Not wanting to tie up an ER bed for something we could treat at home, we felt it was a good idea to get a professional's opinion.

OK, normally on ER and doctor visits one of us will take the hurt or sick child to the ER or doctor's office and one will watch over the other two children. This was the plan in the beginning, and since Lizzy had called in sick and been with Tony all day she said that she'd take him this time. Lizzy knew his symptoms and could convey to the doctor the problem without it being second hand information. Something didn't feel right this time though. I'm not exactly sure what came over me, but when I got home and changed from my work clothes, I found myself calling my brother-in-law and asking him to watch Sam and Zak while we took Tony to the ER. With the tight family we have, Mike was over in less than ten minutes.

A Line That Was Drawn

While driving to the ER, Tony was having more trouble breathing and he was finding it hard to stay awake, which started to frighten us a little more than before. Arriving at the ER, Lizzy went to fill out the appropriate paper work while I sat with my son. Tony slouched in the chair and I was continuing to get more concerned with his every breath, which was becoming a labored effort. I looked up and saw a sign saying if you are having breathing problems let us know right away. We were definitely falling into this category right about now, so I went up and interrupted Lizzy's conversation with the secretary. I told her of Tony's breathing problems. It wasn't sixty seconds later that a nurse was escorting us back to the ER to check his stats. Not that we knew a whole bunch about stats at the time, Tony's blood oxygen level was at 70% when it's supposed to be at least 95%.

After the x-ray and thirty minutes passing the doctor came into the room with a look on his face that still sends chills down my spine. He told us we have a very sick boy on our hands and that an ambulance was on its way to take us to a hospital that was better equipped to handle Tony's severe condition. At this time we were feeling a little uneasy and confused. The Doctor was asking us of underlying conditions with Tony. There are none! He has never had asthma or any kind of breathing problems. No weight issues either. My Tony is a healthy, active, little boy! It's kind of like the seconds after a car crash. You're just in the state of *what the hell just happened?* Ambulance? Better equipped hospital?

They gave us a choice between OU Children's Hospital and a couple of others. There wasn't any thought as to which hospital we wanted to go to, OU Children's Hospital. The nice thing was that it was only half an hour away from the house. Since we'll probably be there overnight at best, it will be a short trip to get Tony back to the house where Lizzy and I have successfully watched over him for the past ten years.

Chapter Six

Lizzy rode in the ambulance with Tony, and I followed in my truck. On the trip to the hospital Tony was still having a hard time staying awake due to his blood oxygen level, but he said he remembered seeing my truck following. Once we arrived at OU medical center Tony, Lizzy and the paramedics waited for me to park the truck and catch up to them before they headed to his room.

On the way up the elevator the paramedic pushed the button for the PICU (Pediatric Intensive Care Unit). Feeling aggravated, I was thinking this guy doesn't know where the hell he's going. We don't need the PICU! We just need a room to monitor Tony for a little while, maybe overnight. Surely that doesn't require the PICU! That's for the really sick kids, not our Tony! Right? It finally dawned on me that the regular rooms were probably on the same floor as the PICU. After breathing a sigh of relief, born of ignorance, we arrived on our floor. Walking down the hall I saw the path to the PICU. We won't be going that way! We'll just keep walking to the "just staying a little while" rooms. But wait, we're turning down the PICU hallway!? NO....NO....NO! This can't be right!

While holding my breath in disbelief, Tony was transferred from the gurney to the bed. The room seemed rather large with the south wall being all windows with a glass door looking to the nurses' station. The west wall had a sink, a door leading to the bathroom and a computer for the nurses. The north wall had one window with a chair that pulled out into a sleeping chair barely big enough for one.

I was still thinking, though, we were in the wrong room of the hospital we'll only be here a short time, so the single chair will be fine for our short stay. The east wall was where Tony was lying. To the right of him was a single pole to hang medications. To the left was the monitor that would reveal his soon-to-be stats. The nurses wasted no time getting Tony all hooked up to the monitor… While doing so we were rushed off to fill out a little required paperwork. The paperwork could have easily been brought to us and filled out in the room. But, I think they did this so the doctors and nurses could do their thing without us getting in the way.

When we came back from filling out the mandatory paperwork, which took about 15 minutes, Tony was all wired up! He had the wires monitoring his pulse, blood pressure and his oxygen level, which was at 75% thanks to the oxygen he was receiving from the tube hanging on the end of his nose. The doctor was not at all happy with 75%, so he said Tony was going to be put on what's called a Bi-Pap machine to help get oxygen through his lungs to his bloodstream. Every time Tony would take a breath the machine would push oxygen into his lungs, and from Tony's response, it was not at all comfortable. For the first 20 minutes he fought the machine, pulling it off every chance he got and crying, saying, "But, Dad, it hurts to breathe this deep!" As any parent knows, what hurts our children hurts us tenfold, and this was breaking our hearts.

Lizzy and I just patiently kept after it, no matter how much it hurt us, saying, "This is what we need to do to get better, Tony." But in the back of my mind I'm thinking we don't need this! All we need is just a little oxygen under his nose for a little while and we'll be fine.

One of the hardest things to do that night was to let go of the reins and allow the doctors and nurses to do their jobs. For Tony's entire life, since childbirth, Lizzy and I have supplied all of his needs! Now we're just supposed to stand back and watch? Surely there's something we can do! We did help out wherever we could, but Tony's well being was no longer in our hands. It was in the hands of strangers wearing scrubs and lab coats, their badge proclaiming, "I belong here and I know what I'm doing." I wasn't convinced. Sure, their movements were direct and purposeful, and they talked like they had done this a million times, but this wasn't just any kid here. This is part of me lying on the table before you. One of the four reasons I enjoy coming home every night. This is my son, my buddy. The one I like to hang out with, to play games with, to go riding four wheelers with, and sometimes to do nothing more than cruise around in the truck with the tunes turned up and chat about whatever comes to mind. This is my pal. Please, oh please be right in your decisions, because I don't have a badge.

Most of the night, we struggled with the idea of hurting Tony in order to help him. When he was finally able to tolerate it enough, he fell asleep. Lizzy and I were able to close our eyes for short periods but never really getting any rest. We would hold our breath with every beep from a monitor and look at each other in disbelief of our circumstance. I would try to assure Lizzy that this was still just a temporary problem and we would probably be out of here in the next few hours. Earlier in the night when I told her this, we both believed it. Instead, my heart started to sink when telling her this again while the feeling of uncertainty started to intrude our room.

While Lizzy and I were chatting and wondering if we would get any real sleep that night, we looked out the window and saw the beautiful rays of the early Oklahoma sunrise. This was our last giggle for weeks. We looked at each other and said, "Well, guess not!"

To end our peacefulness with Tony sleeping and Lizzy and I sharing a little time, a man pushing a mobile x-ray machine entered the room. He said, "This will only take a second, you may leave now."

Leave? I don't think so! The thought of leaving Tony's bedside made me feel sick. The man saw our determination and said, "Fine, but you need to put these vests on to protect yourselves from the x-ray."

No problem! The x-ray did only take a short time and the sliding doors were glass but I just wasn't in the position to be parted from my son.

For the next three hours Tony fell in and out of sleep and his blood oxygen level jumped and dived at the same tempo. It would drop to 70% then climb to 90%. This was all while still on the Bi-Pap machine pushing 100% oxygen. It was concerning me but I had no choice other than to allow my ignorance to blanket and comfort me, for sanities sake.

The nurses were like eagles, if not coming into our room, they were sitting at their desk facing the glass doors able to see Tony's every move and would note his stats coming from the monitor. This was comforting, but we were starting to feel like we were a distressing exhibit in a zoo.

While hovering over Tony, two Lab Coats entered the room. Both Lizzy and I jumped up in anticipation of a hopeful diagnosis. They started the conversation with a timid smile that slowly and painfully dissolved into a look that almost put me to my knees and with good reason. They said that Tony needed to go on a ventilator to better his oxygen level and to give his lungs a break to heal. "We will be putting him to sleep while on this vent. It will be a tube going down his throat to the point where his lungs separate."

The thought of Tony getting some much-needed, restful sleep drew a smile from me, which was quickly painted over with a much darker color when the Lab Coats continued their assault. "Tony has a collapsed lung and will need a chest tube to drain the built-up fluid and air pushing against his chest cavity."

We were now feeling much weaker than before, but they still didn't stop with their brutal attack. They also said there is a strong possibility Tony may need the ECMO (extracorporeal membrane oxygenation) machine. Puzzled and allowing a little anger to cover my sorrow, I hastily asked about the machine. "It's a device used when one's lungs are failing. We would put a catheter into the artery in his thigh. This would be attached to a hose that would draw the blood out of Tony's body. His blood would run through the ECMO, and the ECMO would oxygenate the blood and then be put back into his body with another catheter entering in through the artery in his neck. Your son's lungs are starting to fail, but the implication of the ECMO is only a possibility for now."

They brought consent forms for us to sign and handed us three papers explaining ECMO.

All I could do was sit back down and hold onto Lizzy in hopes that our support system would stay strong between us. I was stripped of the comforting thought on our overnight stay. Our world was starting to crumble around us. To sidestep the pain, I quickly jumped up and said, "Babe, it's time to call in the troops."

We both whipped out our cell phones and started searching for the numbers of our loved ones, letting them know of the situation and pleading for their appearance and prayers.

Chapter Seven

The doctors and nurses started to flood the room. They told us in order to put the chest tube in they needed a sterile environment. Being too unstable to move, his room was about to become a surgical room as well. Gathering that washing my hands wouldn't be sufficient, Lizzy and I hesitantly exited the room. On the way out, I bent down to talk to Tony for a quick second. To my dismay, he was already asleep from the drugs administered into his IV. With a whisper and my hands on his bare chest and shoulder I told him, "Be strong. Mommy and Daddy are going nowhere but outside the glass doors. I love you more than you will ever know, my dear son."

After Lizzy was finished saying her see you laters, we left the room. Our thoughts about hovering in front of the window painfully diminished when the curtains were drawn in order save us from seeing them cut into our child.

"Let's go find some coffee. I need to move. I need to stretch. I need to do something to occupy my mind." I growled.

Lizzy quickly agreed, and in a daze we started to wander the area staying close by to what we later found would be our 34-day home.

While waiting on friends and family to appear, we were wanting to lean on each other for support, trying to find a brighter side to all of this, searching for a glimmer of hope that all was going to be fine. However, trying to lean on each other was like leaning on a standing chain link fence without any bars for support. We were weak from lack of sleep and could think only of our child laying on that bed fighting for every breath.

As our loved ones started to show, a doctor seemed to appear out of thin air. He looked as tired and rundown as we felt. With an uneasy aura surrounding him he said, "We have to put Tony on the ECMO now!"

What was just an hour ago a possibility of ECMO came to a definite... it has to be implemented now! I shrunk 6 inches with that one line from the doctor, and I looked at him and said, "You don't seem too sure of yourself!"

I was thinking, maybe we should we try for another doctor? Minus this man's professional looking hair cut and dry-cleaned lab coat, he looks like he'd already failed before even beginning!

With red-rimmed eyes, he allowed me into his world. "Hugh," he said "this is the line in the sand; this is all we can do to save your child's life."

I felt as though I was going to throw up. Turning to Lizzy and seeing the same in her eyes, I quickly had to force my shoulders back and pick my head up; now was not the time for me to break, it was time for me to support my best friend. After shaking the doctor's hand and watching him drift back into Tony's room, I felt Lizzy crumble in my arms. It was all I could do to support my wife, the one who not so long ago sat beside me on the swing set in the park, chatting and laughing into the night, wondering together what was to come in our future.

A Line That Was Drawn

Two more painful hours had passed when the once beaten down doctor came out of the room with a whole new vibe to him. He now approached us with his head up and a friendly look about him. He said, "Getting Tony hooked up to the vent and ECMO was an errorless success!"

With a slight sigh of relief escaping me we asked if we could see him now. He told us that the nurses were just about finished, it would be just a couple more minutes and yes, you can go back in. Lizzy and I waited, not able to say a word; we gripped each other's hand longing for more time with our son.

As the last nurse started to exit the room, she pulled the curtains back again so all could see into the room through the glass doors. Walking to Tony's bedside I could no longer support my own weight. As I fell to my knees I cried, "OHH MY BABY, MY SON! NO!" For it no longer looked like our Tony! He had the ventilator protruding from his mouth. The hoses for the ECMO machine were taped around his head. I could just barely see his adorable face. There was a tube the size of a pixie stick exiting the right side of his chest. And what was one pole of meds were now two. I knelt there at his bedside for an unknown length of time. The world just seemed to stop. I saw or heard nothing other than Tony and the peculiar barking noises the machines made stating my son was still alive. Somehow finding the strength to stand again I embraced Lizzy. We just held each other crying and staring in disbelief, wondering when we would thankfully awaken from this nightmare.

Through the rest of the evening and into the night all we could do was stare at our son while he silently screamed for help. Our hands were now bound by the doctors and nurses. There was no more communicating with Tony because of the drug-induced coma. There was no more movement from Tony, not even a twitch to ease or minds. This was because of the paralytics keeping him still. If he were to move during this stage the catheter entering into his jugular vein in his neck could dislodge and he would bleed out in a matter of seconds.

I pulled one of the doctors to the side wanting to know a little more about Tony's condition. I asked him if we were dealing with the dreaded H1N1. He told me Tony's lab tests were sent off to the CDC, and since they were so backed up it would take weeks to get the results. He also said that almost all Type "A" influenza tests were being considered as the H1N1, and Tony had tested positive for type "A". However the results of these tests would have no bearing on Tony's treatment, as all strains of influenza are treated the same.

Tony had been on the ECMO and vent for over 24 hours when my father in-law, Dennis, who had come up from Tyler asked us, "When was the last time you ate?" Lizzy and I looked at each other and wondered, but couldn't remember. We didn't feel hungry. It would have been a waste of time to tell Dennis we weren't going to eat anything. He said, "Go and get something to eat and try to get a nap in at the very least. I'll stay and keep an eye on Tony. I'll call your cell if anything happens."

Abandoning Tony was not real high on our to-do list, but a bite to eat started to sound like a good way to direct our thoughts to something lighter. Still thinking about Tony, we found ourselves in the cafeteria wondering how we'd tell Samantha and Zak. We decided we'd tell them tomorrow night, and be straight with them, like we always have. We couldn't find any reason not to tell the kids exactly what was going on with their Bobo, as Zak called him. It would have been easier to say that he just has the flu and everything was going to be fine. But my gut was reminding me of my uncertainty. The very thought of telling the kids what was going on had me feeling sick to my stomach. Telling our kids would make this more of a reality. Our kids learn not only by what they're told, but by what they see. So it was time again to hold my head up put my shoulders back and help them face our nightmare Together.

After eating, the idea of getting some sleep was starting to sound better all the time. We decided we would take turns taking catnaps in the room with Tony. While counting tiles on the floor on our way back to Tony's room, we looked up just before entering and were stopped by a stranger. A man wearing a black suit with a white collar patiently waited for our attention.

I immediately thought the worst. I bolted for the door and saw a loving man sitting next to the bed looking up to give me a humble smile. Oh thank GOD! Everything is OK! Tony's stats are the same as before. So I turned and saw the man was still standing there, now with his hand outreached wanting me to do the same. I looked at him and said, "OH NO, MISTER! I'M NOT READY TO BE TALKING TO YOU RIGHT NOW!" The thought of a chaplain wanting to speak with us now directed my thought process in a direction I wasn't willing to go.

My thought was that the chaplain always showed up in the moment most needed, at or towards the end of a loved one's life. I was becoming so heartbroken that it would have been real easy to turn it into anger and direct it all towards the innocent man standing before me. I just shook my head and stormed off feeling as though it was the Grim Reaper himself wanting to have a conversation. I'll have no part in that!

Before I could push the bar on the PICU exit door, I felt the man turning his attention towards Lizzy. I could just feel it. I turned to see Lizzy standing in front of the chaplain using all her strength to keep her composure. I felt as though she was overwhelmed by it all and wasn't able to say no if she wanted to. To make sure of my feelings, I went to her and said, "If you don't want to talk with this man, don't."

Being married for 11 years does have its advantages, and this time it was like I could feel Liz screaming at me for help; and me just waiting for any man bold enough to touch the chip on my shoulder. I'm still not certain if she wanted to talk with him or she saw the fury in my eyes, but she just turned, opened the glass doors to our son's room and entered, gracefully shutting the door behind her.

Knowing in the back of my mind this man's intentions were pure; I turned my attention to him and said, "Look buddy, I'm holding on to sanity by not much more than a string here." Trying to calm myself a little before I continued, I said, "You're probably going to help us about as much as God is right now, so we don't want to talk to you."

To my surprise, he responded in a fashion I wasn't prepared for. He looked at me through the most gentle of eyes and with compassion in his voice he said, "Maybe you should give that string to God." I needed to release all the frustration building up inside and ask God "why all this was happening;" I instead hardened myself and bolted for the exit. I had no idea at the time what God was up to, but He did.

Throughout the rest of the night we took turns resting and shutting our eyes in the big blue chair. We were never really able to sleep with the nurses coming in and out every 15 minutes to check on Tony. And the machines continued to inform us that our son was still alive. We were overly exhausted, but the very idea of Tony's condition robbed us from any sleep that night.

A Line That Was Drawn

During the night while talking with one of the nurses, I started to realize how difficult their job was. They endured twelve-hour shifts and breaks were determined by their patients' current status. They started to ask questions about who my boy was and what he liked to do. They also asked what he looked like before being in this situation. The nurse wanted to see some pictures of Tony doing the things he loved. They recommended we decorate the room a little.

Within a couple of days, our dear friend, Leslie, went by our house and retrieved some pictures for us to hang around the room. We placed some pictures of Tony above his headboard in between the oxygen hookups and the nurses call button. It wasn't long after this that Tony's teacher, Mrs. Pezant, brought up get-well cards made by his classmates. These were hung on the west wall along with the card made by Tony's best buddy, Chris. Earlier, when Chris came to visit and deliver his card, he needed help standing while seeing his buddy in this condition.

Seeing the nurses' reaction to Tony's pictures and cards made me wonder. They all enjoyed the newly decorated room and appreciated having his pictures above his bed. They now could put a face to the figure lying before them. I wondered how they could do their job without getting too emotionally attached. Working as a nurse in a hospital is one thing, but working with ailing children in a PICU takes a special type of person.

I have a job. In-between Friday afternoon and Monday morning, I don't think about this job. This gives me time to recoup for the next week. Acquiring a position at a PICU is not a job, but a way of life. I mean really, how do you forget about a child you've been working on all week and resume life outside these walls with a clear head? The staff that works at OU Pediatric Intensive Care Unit is the elite in their field.

Chapter Eight

The x-ray tech entered with the sunrise advertising that it was going to be a new and good day. We had a hard time lifting our heads up in agreement. I didn't feel defeated, I just felt like I was in the 3rd round of a boxing match with Mike Tyson and not holding my own very well. Looking into Lizzy's eyes I could tell the feeling was mutual. It was like being backed over by a truck and still able to limp away.

After the x-ray tech left, we were told the doctors will be making their rounds in a little while and will update us on Tony's prognosis. This was told to us in a casual manner, but we took it as the end all of conversations for the day. Whenever we heard "they're making rounds," nothing was more important. Not breakfast, friends or family would keep us from peering out the glass doors nervously awaiting our moment with the Attending Physician... This became part of our daily routine for our stay at OU Children's.

This morning was important, because we thought we were long overdue for some good news. His stats were up and his oxygen levels were at satisfactory levels. As the Attending Physician entered the room, Lizzy and I held our breath in anticipation for good news. The Attending agreed with us about the stats and oxygen levels, but said it was due to the ECMO machine. Tony may look better on the monitors, but looking at the x-ray, his condition was *worsening*. His lung was not only collapsing but it was also snow white on the x-ray; while his other lung shows black which is a clear airway. The Attending was not looking positive at this point. I struggled to find a bit of hopefulness in his voice or even demeanor. But I received not even a hint of good news. Tony's outlook was not good. The doctors remained hopeful, but I could see the grim outlook in their eyes. When they and the nurses passed our room I could see it; Hopeful yes, but this day we were being looked at with sympathetic eyes. They didn't have to say a thing. I could tell by the way they looked at us; we were losing the battle.

    We arranged with my brother in-law, Mike, and my sister, Lorie, to have them bring up Samantha and Zak later that afternoon. The kids had been staying with them for the time being. I had been preparing myself all day for the time with our children. Not just to break the news, but to hold onto them as tightly as they would allow me. Samantha unknowingly holds my heart in hers, and with mine breaking right now, I longed to look in those big brown eyes of innocence to entice hope and courage. Samantha and I have had a relationship only a father could know or understand. She can set my soul at ease and calm my spirit with just a glance. She can brighten my day with just a simple "HI DADDY!"

    When they arrived at the hospital it was a heartfelt reunion. It had been only two days since we saw them last but it felt like weeks. We needed a quiet place so Lizzy and I could talk to the kids without interruption. I saw a sign for the chapel on the 3rd floor saying the doors were never locked. This would be appropriate and would do fine.

To my relief, the room was empty. Lizzy and the kids followed me to the front row of the pews. While walking towards the front I thankfully saw a large cross. It humbled and supported me. Lizzy and the kids sat on the front pew, while I knelt in front of them. We just laid it on the line, there would be no beating around the bush; this is what's going on with your BoBo. We didn't go into details about the machines thinking that might make things a little confusing. We told them of the severity of Tony's condition, and were able to get all the words out until... While we were explaining, it sunk in a little with Samantha and I looked into her eyes and saw the pain in her as though it were a mirror image of mine. I could no longer be the big strong dad I was taught to be by my own dad; all I could do was wrap my family in my arms. There was no strength left in me to sustain.

While our family was having the chance to mourn the situation together, Zakery broke free from the family hug and with tears pouring down his face, said, "Don't worry, Daddy, Tony's not going to die!" Never once did we say anything about dying, but he seemed to know something we didn't. He said it the same way he says, *"This toy is mine!"* totally sure of what he was saying was the absolute truth. After falling back into my arms, I felt a tremendous peace blanket us. I think there were angels there not to just guide and comfort us, but also to send a message through Zakery.

After seeing that the kids were starting to bounce back a little, still somber but able to communicate, we took them to Tony's room. We stood outside the doors looking at our BoBo, holding onto one another still in disbelief. That's when Zakery put my feelings into action. Gotta move, talk, stretch, run, and play, just anything but stand here! Lizzy and I agreed it was time for some Samantha and Zak time, playing games and having a little fun to redirect their innocent minds. We went to the family room where we found some cards and blocks supplied by my buddy, Steve, and his mother, Pam. It was hard to join in playing with the kids, while thinking I needed to go and hover over Tony, but right now Sam and Zak need us so this is where we'll stay for now.

After a couple of hours Samantha and Zak were starting to get tired, so we said our good-byes and my brother-in-law, Mike, took the kids home with him. Feeling like a car running out of gas, Lizzy and I returned to Tony's room.

That night we each took turns sleeping in the big blue chair while the other monitored Tony. Since we could only sleep for an hour or two at a time, this worked well.

Chapter Nine

The next morning, a little while after Tony's x-ray, the Attending came in. He told us that Tony's x-rays were starting to clear up a little! What had been snow white was now showing a slight bit of clarity. Wow! Finally some good news! He said they were going to start to wean the ECMO a little at a time and see how Tony's oxygen levels hold up. They started with reducing the ECMO to 90%.

Through the next four hours Tony's levels stayed strong! We were told that he would be on a four-hour wean. Every four hours they would take it down another 10%, assuming Tony's stats were stable.

By the next morning the ECMO was as low as it could safely operate. The doctors told us it was time to take him off the ECMO! Lizzy and I felt our nightmare coming to an end. It was like hiking through a dark cave for days and finally being able to see a light far in the distance. We knew we weren't in the clear yet, but at least we were starting to go in the right direction. Finally!

As the surgeons once again shut the door and curtains, Lizzy and I had some bounce back in our step while we walked to the cafeteria. Seeing hope return to Lizzy's eyes again put me at ease and let me know our support system was once again gaining strength. We enjoyed our time alone together without the constant worry of Tony's condition. Tony was in good hands, and besides a leisurely breakfast was long overdue. Even a long awaited smile slipped in from time to time. It had been so long it almost hurt to grin. We were excited to go back up to Tony's room and see him with less hardware entering and surrounding him. Pushing the elevator button five extra times did us absolutely no good. Patience would have to wait until our son was well again. Seeing the door to the stairwell I looked at Lizzy, smiled, and said "Race ya!" We arrived at Tony's room completely out of breath.

After the surgeons were finished and seeing their crew leaving with smiles on their faces, we reentered Tony's room. It was really cool to be able to see Tony's face again! There was no longer tape holding the ECMO hoses to his face. We could recognize our son for the first time in five days. What a relief, we were getting or son back! They would remind us the battle wasn't over, but yes, he was on the road to recovery.

Lizzy and I wondered if people in Oklahoma knew of the severity of getting the H1N1. Seeing that Tony was on a satisfactory trend, our thoughts and worries started to spread to other parents and kids who could be in this horrific situation.

I had to weigh the pros and cons with the decision to go public or not. On one hand, people need to know the complications that can come with the H1N1. People need to know the speed at which things can escalate and how to act appropriately. We want people to know that this flu can no longer be treated like we used to. In the past we would get a hot toddy and a trash bag sitting readily next to our bed, and in a couple of days everything would be fine. We wanted to let people know we could no longer treat the flu in this manner. We wanted to scream it from the rooftops, if you're having breathing problems associated with the flu, it's time to go to the doctor's office. And if you can't get immediate attention there, go to the ER.

On the other hand, if my voice became too loud and penetrating, there could be a mad frenzy at the medical centers. The lines could get so long the kid in front of the line could be there with his frantic parents over a harmless cough, while the kid at the end of the line was in need of some serious medical attention.

In making a decision of this magnitude, I started to seek out advice from people much smarter than I. Speaking with Attendings, nurses and family members. Everybody saw the potential problems of either decision I made. After pondering and talking with people for a couple of hours I made my decision.

I decided that informing people of the situation on our hands was the best way to fight it. My hope was that people would act rationally and appropriately, just so long as they would act if needed.

Since my father, John, had worked at KFOR channel 4 for over thirty-five years, they were the only ones I thought of calling. While on the phone with the KFOR operator, she forwarded me to the newsroom where I spoke to someone about our story and our need to let people know of the severity. They told me someone would be calling me back shortly.

Not ten minutes later my phone rang, and to my surprise it was one of my favorite newscasters in the business, Meg Alexander. I gave a brief run down and she said she wanted to come interview us. I told her that would be fine and I'll see you soon.

Telling Lizzy this didn't have the outcome I had expected. We had our chance to warn Oklahomans and possibly save some lives with our information. She said, "Oh no, I'm not standing in front of a camera and talking!" She never has been the spotlight type of gal. She's the type who works behind the scenes and is content to do so. Her being the brains of the family and me being the guy who likes flying blindly at times, we planned what we thought needed to be told.

An hour had passed when my phone rang again, this time it was from the Public Relations department, Allen, representing OU Children's Hospital. He would set up the meet and wanted to make sure I was ok with everything. He was our knight standing guard, not allowing anybody to speak to us or see us in the hospital without going through him first. From then on I've had much respect for this model of a man.

Preceding the interview, I wondered if I could hold it together while speaking to Oklahoma about my son. Deciding that our message was much bigger than me, I became content with my intended demeanor in front of the camera.

The interview with Meg went smooth; Meg was sympathetic and understanding of our situation. With Meg being a parent herself, it wasn't long before a change arose. The interview started with a reporter and a story, but following the interview after the story was told and the camera was shut off, things between Meg and I changed. I was no longer a story and she was no longer a reporter. We were two parents struggling to comprehend the impact this virus was going to have on our great state and nation. Saying our goodbyes, Meg hugged me in a way only a good friend could have. It was then I knew she fully understood and shared in the heartache.

A reporter by the name of Linda Mares was next to take our story. Little did I know at the time she would be with us throughout our stay. Linda would call me two or three times a week just to see how we were holding up, partly for the story but mostly to lend an ear of understanding and support. I've never known the media to be so personable, yet I was thankful for the sociability from Linda.

This was followed by many more interviews, including the national spotlight with Katie Couric. Thankfully, our warning seemed to snowball with the media all going through Allen, our modern day Knight. (Some of these interviews can be found on my website.)

While happy with the information we were able to convey, I could now direct all of my attention back to Tony. Today they were going to start reducing Tony's paralytics, yet another sign he was on the road to recovery! At 2:00 p.m. the paralytics were reduced to 50%. This was allowing him to start coughing up all the junk built up in his lungs. While being totally sedated he wasn't able to cough, so they would suction through his breathing tube to simulate a cough. This was doing a fair job but not as well as a real cough. I've never been so happy to see mucus in my life! He was coughing up loads. Even though he was coughing now, he was still heavily sedated and only opened his eyes a sliver from time to time. For now, that was all we needed to gratefully smile.

Sleep seemed to be determined by our comfort level; and on that Monday afternoon we both napped peacefully, Comforted by the thought that our Tony would be up and moving again in the next couple of days. That night Lizzy and I were still keeping our guard up, and taking turns sleeping at his bedside. While the other stayed awake updating friends and family by means of texts, Lizzy's MySpace page and Facebook sites.

About 2:00 a.m. Lizzy abruptly woke me and said, "You need to get up, there is something wrong with Tony!" Wiping the sleep from my eyes, I was horrified to see Tony's blood oxygen level at 60%! When I fell asleep just a couple of hours ago he was a solid 94%! What's going on? All we could do is stand back and watch the room flood with doctors and nurses accompanied with the returning horror we thought we had conquered just yesterday. While I felt the blood drain from my face, I looked at Lizzy seeking the assurance that everything was going to be OK, that this was just a hiccup and will soon pass. But I only saw what I was too feeling, sheer terror!

Tony's oxygen level was now dipping into the 50's. Seeing this, the Attending quickly took Tony off the vent and bagged him calmly saying, "We've got to get more oxygen into this little boy now!" Lizzy's and my fears could not have been any higher, we couldn't move and we had a hard time catching our breath. I thought my knees were going to buckle when we heard the Attending say, "I'm not losing one tonight!" No longer in the calm voice we had grown used to. Tony's oxygen levels were now dropping to 30%.

My hand began to hurt with Lizzy's clamp on mine. OH GOD NO! This can't be it! Can it? Is this the time to interrupt the doctors so I can say goodbye to our son? None of the staff was giving up, but occasionally I would catch a glimpse of one of the nurses glancing at me with sympathetic eyes. It was though they wanted to prepare for the worst and wondered how we would react.

Bagging Tony was going on for two painful hours now. The Attending was trying everything she could, fearfully not squeezing the air bag too hard, because that could result in overinflating and popping Tony's lungs. But we had to get his oxygen level up! It was a fine line of hard enough to get oxygen in the good lung but not so hard to pop it. She would peer at us frequently and then hurry and get back to work. Tony was showing no progress.

Then finally the Attending said, "Let's flip him!" Without any questions, the nurses enthusiastically responded by preparing all the wires and hoses for the flip. Now Tony was lying on his stomach, nothing changed in the way they were treating him. The bag was still being rapidly compressed when his oxygen level started to climb. "We're at 50%, come on, Tony," the Attending murmured. "You can do it! Come on, Tony!" Up to 60% and still rising! We plateaued at a bone chilling 70% when the Attending said to put him back on the vent with 100% oxygen. We remained between 70 and 80% for the rest of the night and into the daylight hours.

After the x-ray tech was finished taking pictures and the doctors had time to review them, the order came to switch Tony's vent to an oscillator. To us, not being in the medical field, it was one of the scariest of machines. It would almost fully inflate Tony's lungs and keep them there, only offering rapid shallow breaths while inflated; Kind of like a dog panting on a hot summer day. Though it may look scary the doctor advised that this would be the easiest pressure on Tony's lungs. We were beside ourselves with dismay.

"Since we're not for certain why your son took such a sudden and tremendous dive last night, we want to do a CT scan of his lungs."

We were all for the doctors arming themselves with as much information as possible. My thoughts were, you have to find the cause before finding a cure.

Chapter Ten

After filling out the paperwork that was needed, they scheduled a time to get Tony into the CT. I had no idea what would be involved in transporting Tony to the CT. What a feat it was! His meds and monitor had to become mobile. He was also taken off the vent and bagged. This was a six-person job including Lizzy and I. We may not have an education that constitutes a degree but my son was traveling on a gurney now and needed a direct path to the CT room. I'm just the guy needed to clear a path or an elevator. Because of Tony being contagious, we had to don full masks and temporary scrubs. Walking down the halls in this manner, with people in the way, it didn't take long for them to move when hearing "H1N1 contagious boy coming through!"

The journey to and from the CT went without a hitch; it was while laying on the CT table problems arose. His blood pressure rose to scary heights while his blood oxygen level dipped back into the 60s. Thankfully there were oxygen hookups in the room. This was Tony's way of telling us he didn't want to be moved!

Shortly after our endeavor, the Attending approached us saying in a gentle voice, "I would like to talk to the both of you and go over the results from the CT scan."

Lizzy and I quickly arose from Tony's bedside and followed the Attending. After he abruptly cleared the viewing room of all doctors and nurses, he positioned the chairs so we could sit in a good viewing area in front of the large computer monitors. After taking a deep breath, he pulled up Tony's CT scan. With a CT scan you can take the picture and cut it horizontally to view the organ in slices. In doing so the Attending showed us a lung that was so infected there was no air present to say the least. The lung was now solid white with infection. *Tony was worse off now than he was after arriving a week ago.* I continually asked questions as to how, why, and what? This just can't be! He was doing great just a day and a half ago.

The Attending continued his ambush on our very being. He said, "Even if we are able to identify and successfully fight this, there remains the grave possibility of scar tissue." He continued to say, "With too much scar tissue in one's lung, the lung can no longer function."

I repeated my previous questions of how, why and what! He just humbly repeated his answers waiting for this to sink in with us. Staring at the pictures a little longer, I felt my heart start to melt. My body wanted to give way to the increased gravity. Tears were welling up in my eyes when I unknowingly shouted, "I've got to go!"

While looking at the Attending on the way out I noticed that that his eyes were full of remorse. I sure didn't need to see that! Somehow making it to Tony's doors, peering in at him, I felt a hand grasp mine. It was my best friend, Lizzy. I turned to her and held on to her as though our life depended on it. Sanity was becoming but a dream I had long ago. I felt myself slipping away thinking, *I don't think I can take much more of this.*

Feeling eyes on us, we broke our embrace to turn and see who was watching us. It just so happened to be the only men in my life who could keep me grounded; my dad, John, and Lizzy's dad, Dennis. Seeing them, I could finally allow myself to crumble, knowing my dad would be where he has always been; ready to pick me up whenever I fell. There were no questions, he just looked at me shaking his head and with his arms stretched open he said, "NO!" Being a 37-year-old man standing at 6'2" I was able to regress to simpler times, preteen, needing to be held by the man who wanted nothing more from me than what I wanted from my own son. This is My Daddy. I feel safe now, if only for a moment.

After I regained some composure the Attending approached me saying, "I've got an idea." I quickly followed him to an unoccupied room. He told me there was this drug that they use for premature babies. The drug was used to open the air sacks in a baby's lungs. Since the baby wasn't supposed to be born yet, the chemical the body produces to open air sacks in the lungs hasn't been produced yet. He told me they had the drug on hand but it's expensive.

I asked, "Do you think this could help Tony?"

He said he couldn't be certain, but it was worth a shot. After finding out the price tag on one dose, (around $10,000) I wasn't for sure if insurance would cover the cost or not, I told him, "We'll take five doses!"

He chuckled a little and said, "Hugh, we'll start with one maybe two doses and see where that gets us."

Not wasting any time, he ordered the drug and administered it into Tony's IV. About an hour later I started searching for the Attending. After finding him, I asked if he would check on Tony to see if the drug was working. I felt a little hope slip away when he told me it would be at least a week to see any results.

Dragging myself back to Tony's room, I saw Lizzy sitting in the room. When I put on my mask and gown to enter the room, Lizzy gave me a little card she had gotten from the gift shop downstairs, the size of a business card, Lizzy's eyes were watery. She said, "I need some air."

Pulling a chair up next to Tony's bed I read the card to myself at first and thought this is perfect. I read it again, this time aloud to Tony. It said, "I Am Special, I Am Strong and I Can Do Anything!" I said it to him again, "I Am Special, I Am Strong and I Can Do Anything!" Then I said it to him again, "I Am Special, I Am Strong and I Can Do Anything!" I told him, "Tony, I am not telling you who you are; I am reminding you of who you are now! You Are Strong, You Are Special and You, my son, Can Do Anything!"

I continued talking to Tony about everything going on, from the people who had come to visit him to the weather outside. I had to stop frequently to stop my voice from cracking. If I was reminding him to be strong then I must lead by example.

Seeing a book that had been read to me when I was in 5th grade by my all-time favorite teacher, Mrs. Lowman, I picked it up and began to read "Summer Of The Monkeys." My brother in-law, Tony, and sister, Mandy, had brought it up on my request the day before.

While switching back and forth from reading to just talking then back to reading again, Tony's blood pressure started to rise. Not just too elevated heights, but to the point where it set off the alarm that alerted the nurses. While trying to find out the problem with Tony's blood pressure, they administered a drug into his IV to bring it down to a satisfactory level. Lizzy entered the room at this time. The nurses, not being comfortable with the results from the blood pressure medication, quickly ran off to get the Attending. That's when Lizzy had an idea that I will be thankful for, for the rest of my life. She pulled out a CD and put it in the CD player. It was Tony's favorite singer, Carrie Underwood. As that angelic voice filled the room, I looked in amazement as Tony's blood pressure slowly started to subside. We turned Carrie up a little more to see Tony's blood pressure drop to a, once again, comfortable level.

For the rest of our stay, anytime we had a problem with Tony's pressures you could hear Carrie singing "Jesus, Take The Wheel" and many others. Her heartfelt songs inspired us. Carrie unknowingly bought us time to allow Tony's lung to heal. I hope to meet Carrie someday, not for an autograph or to meet a superstar, but to wrap my arms around her and thank her for being an angel who shed light on our darkest days.

Chapter Eleven

Feeling relieved from yet another crisis, I had to stretch my legs. While passing the nurses' station I saw one of the Attendings sitting down concentrating deeply on her work, so I wouldn't interrupt her thoughts. As she looked up, I simply smiled and said, "Hi."

She broke her concentration to talk to me. "Hugh, there's a possibility we can get Tony back on the ECMO!"

Knowing that Tony's lungs needed a break to heal I told her, "I read in the paperwork from the previous ECMO induction, that it was a onetime deal, after one got off it you could never go back on again?"

She said, "It depends on the condition of the entry point on the vein. We are discussing getting an ultrasound of the injection point to see if it's possible." Seeing the excitement starting to rise in me, she quickly reminded me, "This is only a possibility."

Ignoring that last little tidbit, I ran to find Lizzy and tell her the news. In the back of my mind knowing it was only a "possibility" of the induction, we couldn't help but to grasp the little bit of hope before us. While discussing the possibilities, we thought, *WOW, Round Two.* "We're starting all over again, babe."

While hovering over Tony, a lady entered the room with a machine not seen since looking at our unborn children. The ultrasound had arrived. The tech was trying to do her job and ignoring my many questions in order to do so. My mouth seemed to try and match my nerves, going a hundred miles per hour at this point.

About an hour after the ultrasound tech was finished, we started seeing doctors congregate outside our room. When there seemed to be enough staff to work on a small city, one of the most familiar faces, our Attending, entered the room. He said the surgeons felt comfortable with the condition of the vein, and saw it as a good possibility they would be successful. When the eyes outside the doorway saw our heads nod, they took that as the signal to commence. While trading places with the many surgeons, attending physicians and nurses, Tony's room was once more transformed into a sterile operating room. Seeing the curtains close again, we waited.

It took them about an hour this time to get Tony hooked up to the ECMO once again. We felt relieved to see them coming out with a content look on their faces. Once more Tony's face was covered by hoses attached with tape. A little more recognizable this time due to them cutting back on the tape and turning his head to the other side towards the window.

While looking at Tony I had to keep reminding myself, this is Round Two, we've got a lot more fight in us, right Tony? Now bending to talk to my son who was in a drug-induced coma, "Tony, we always have a little more fight left. You just have to dig deep. When you don't think you have anything left, search deep in your gut because it's there, Tony! It's there!"

Looking up I saw our Attending patiently waiting outside the glass doors. Peeling myself away from Tony to talk to the doctor and allow Lizzy to have some time alone with our son, I left the room. He said he found, through a lab test, a *staph* infection out of Tony's IV. It wasn't long after that conversation that we found the *staph* had infected his bloodstream resulting in his lungs being attacked first, due to their weakness from fighting the H1N1. The white we saw on the x-ray was from the severe case of pneumonia.

At the time our doctor wasn't 100% sure which one of the reasons Tony was hitting all time lows. "So," he said, "I'm going to try and treat both possibilities. For the *staph* infection and pneumonia I want to start on the lab's recommendation of antibiotics. There will be three different kinds of antibiotics that will be administered intravenously. These were proven to fight the bacteria successfully in the lab. Also, there is an experimental drug I've been researching called Zanamivir. While being FDA approved for the inhalant form, it has not yet been approved for intravenous application yet. And since Tony is not able to inhale it at this time, due to being in a drug-induced coma, we would have to take the experimental approach. There have been successful applications in other countries."

While talking to Lizzy about this, it started to hit me that now was the time the doctors were reaching, searching for anything that would save our son's life. We no longer had the luxury of uniformed responses to Tony's conditions. The doctors were in unfamiliar territory. I enjoyed watching the doctor's ability to overcome their anxiety of uncertainty and blossom with the idea of the challenge at hand. I guess you don't get to be an Attending at OU Children's PICU by having your name randomly drawn from a hat.

It didn't take Lizzy and I long to make our decision on the experimental drug. All that was needed to get the ball rolling was the required paperwork signed and notarized. Leave it to a hospital of this caliber to have a notary on hand.

Being experimental, the drug was nowhere nearby that he could find at first; the doctor said he may have to get it flown in from Europe. I asked if I could be of any assistance, I told him I'd be willing to fly or drive anywhere needed to obtain this drug and hopefully speed up the process. He gave me a comforting grin and said he'll look into the possibilities. An hour went by when he found the drug here in the States and said it could be here as early as tonight, tomorrow afternoon at the latest.

The experimental drug arrived the following afternoon. Willing to grasp a hold of any kind of hope, Lizzy and I sighed with relief. We were told the first dose would be administered at 9:00 p.m. and be followed every 12 hours for the next five days. This appeared to be the last chance of healing Tony.

Through the night and the next day Tony was up and down with his stats. We were continually bouncing back and forth from the stereo to having our backs to the wall, allowing the nurses to accommodate Tony. Only sleeping in shifts was starting to wear on us, but the frequent adrenaline rushes instigated by Tony were enough to keep us going.

After having a couple of doses of what we hoped was going to be the miracle drug, our Attending came to us with a look that forced me to find a seat. He said, "I'm not certain that this drug is going to be doing Tony any good. We ordered the drug hoping we were dealing mainly with the H1N1. But getting more information from the lab and looking at the x-rays from this morning, our primary focus is the *staph* infection and pneumonia that has attacked Tony's lung, this looks to be the main reason his lung is failing. Also, his lung has collapsed again. We need to put in a larger chest tube because the one in there now seems to be too small to drain the thick puss from the infection collapsing his lung."

With this conversation, we were feeling all hope diminish. Our hearts dropped to the pits of our stomachs. Thinking I couldn't take anymore, the Attending wasn't finished.

He then told us that Tony's kidneys couldn't keep up and needed to go on dialysis. I took that as his body was starting to shut down getting ready for his final exit. Before, I was holding on to sanity by a thread, now I began to feel the string starting to break.

"Hugh and Lizzy," he concluded, "there is nothing more we can do for Tony. We have done all we can. We are out of options here."

Chapter Twelve

Trying to accept the facts, I had to talk to Tony, alone. After the room was clear of everybody, I pulled up a chair next to him getting as close as I could. I wanted to lie in bed with him but the extensive hoses and machines wouldn't allow it. While putting my hand on his forehead and my other hand on his bare chest, I longed to be touching him more. Saying good-bye to my son was something my heart couldn't prepare for, but I didn't want him to leave me without saying how much I adored having him as my son. I had to talk to him about the things he was never able to experience in life. Like what it's like to catch a fish that almost pulls you into the lake. What it's like having your first kiss with a girl you've been dreaming about. What it's like to ride a motorcycle through the Rockies on a warm summer afternoon. What it's like to climb the highest peaks in Colorado. What it's like to walk down the aisle and hear your best friend, your soul mate, say, "I do."

The nurses came in to hook Tony up to the dialysis machine. Lizzy entered the room with them. I told Lizzy, "I've got to take a walk, I'll be back soon." With a desperate hug and what I felt might be my last look at my buddy, I left.

On the way down the elevator, I felt my blood start to boil! My body was starting to tense. My teeth were starting to chatter uncontrollably. My hands started to hurt from being balled so tight. I had to find the reason we were in this situation! Where did he get this? Could it be Scouts, school or football? I couldn't pinpoint it; he could have gotten it anywhere. Did Lizzy put him in a situation to get exposed or did I not bundle him up properly going to the track? We can't live in a bubble! Did family or friends know they were sick and come over and play with Tony anyway? There was nothing to support that argument either.

Once on the first floor and able to see the doors exiting to the outside, for a split second, everything stopped. The sound of my footsteps, my shaking and my hearing all stopped for a just a moment. I had figured it all out! The reason Tony was upstairs fighting for his life. The reason Lizzy and I were sobbing uncontrollably. The reason all of this was going on! Everything burst alive again. I felt like a volcano on the brink of blowing its top! The doors are right in front of me. I've got to go now! It's time, and I'm ready for battle! Knock down drag out don't care if I survive fight! I sprinted for the doors and crashed into them knowing they were sliding, but I didn't care! Nothing mattered now, because I've figured it all out and was ready to go to war with the one who deserved all of the blame! What Tony was going through, what my entire family was struggling to get through, and for what reason? I ran to a place I knew I could be one on one with the conniving culprit. I found my battleground, stood in the middle like I would in a boxing ring, taunting, and waited for him to show!

A Line That Was Drawn

This is all GOD'S fault!!!

Never did I think I would be blaming God for the things going wrong in my life. But hey, this is my son we're talking about here. We have been on local and national news, so I couldn't even imagine how many people were praying for Tony. With that many people praying, how could He not know what was going on? And if He did know, what is He waiting for? Why has He not intervened? Saved at the age of nine and being raised in a Southern Baptist church, my belief in God through Jesus Christ has always been a part of my life, so I thought. Looking back through the years I felt God was God. Not a friend or companion, but the great spirit in the sky that created us. Separate from us on the grandest of pedestals. Deservedly so, no doubt, but, how do I relate? And, how can I expect the ultimate to even care about something like this in my life with all the other things happening in this world? I'm a simple man with simple needs, and up until now I've never really ran into anything in life I couldn't remedy, fix or throw away and get a new one. My belief that Christ lived, never a doubt! But, My belief IN Christ - almost nonexistent. Until this moment I never knew there was a difference. But the difference is night and day. Not having a personal relationship with my Creator and not knowing the extent to which He cares about *everything* in our lives. It was easy to point the finger in His direction and place all the blame on Him. I want you to understand that my heart was in pieces. I felt this world slipping away and didn't care what happened. Sanity was but a dream I had years before. God will not put on us more than we can stand, but I've taken all I can take! It's On!

Shaking my fist at the heavens I prayed, "HOW DARE YOU TRY TO TAKE MY CHILD, HOW DARE YOU!" Completely enraged at the very idea I continued, "COME

DOWN HERE AND FACE ME! LET US END THIS RIGHT HERE AND RIGHT NOW! COME AND FACE ME LIKE A MAN! I'M READY!"

Feeling overwhelmed with outrage I fell to my knees. "I need him more than you do, God! I want him more than you do! He's mine, if you're not going to help, can't you just leave us alone!" For the first time in my life, I wanted nothing to do with the One who blessed me with this child, who I adore. And then turn around 10 years later and steal him from me? How sick is that!?

After a while of sitting there thinking, I picked myself up and sauntered towards Tony's room. Seeing him attached now to a dialysis machine and having four poles of medications, I needed to talk to someone in their right mind. Someone who was strong, someone who wouldn't sugar coat what I needed to hear. I needed to talk to someone who could tell me why God hasn't been present through any of this! I needed someone to tell me why my God was standing on the sidelines when my need for Him has never been greater! I called the strongest man I ever met in my life, one who doesn't sway in his beliefs, the one person I know who stands his ground no matter what the cost or ridicule. Thankfully, my brother John answered the phone. "John," I said, "I need your help."

Discussing with John where I thought the blame should lie, he asked me one simple question. "What decision has God ever made that turned out to be a mistake?" Knowing that it would be a losing battle to try and argue this with John, I hung up the phone and stewed on that thought for awhile.

Could His decision be perfect while taking our son? That was a hard pill to swallow. "GOD, what's happening here?" While praying this, a thought came to mind and a peace I have never felt washed over me. The thought was JESUS CHRIST and what GOD must have felt allowing Him to be brutally crucified on that cross. This decision was, I'm sure, painful but could not have been any more perfect. If He could send his only Son to His death, his decision would be perfect with my son's outcome. His decision is perfect.

Experiencing the peace I felt that night has changed me forever. I was no longer concerned with the reason Tony got sick even though I was still heartbroken by the thought that I could lose my son tonight, but I now knew who held the reins and who was in total control. Knowing this ended my battle with GOD. Giving up what I wanted most and offering my child into His capable hands, was the hardest thing I've ever done. It was finally my time to stop believing solely in God's existence, and come to the understanding that this is what it is to believe IN Him.

Feeling absolutely drained, I had to get some sleep. Tony was not doing so well. His oxygen levels were in the high seventies and that's with the ECMO being at 100%. Also the vent was pushing 100% oxygen. His body wasn't responding to any of the doctor's treatments. So I could be easily awoken, I pulled a chair as close as I could to Tony's bed and laid my hand on his chest. Lying there staring at Tony and praying I said, "God, I put Tony is in your hands now, if you allow us to keep Tony or if your decision is to take my son, I will thank you. Your decision is perfect." The peace that enveloped me after this prayer left no room for uncertainty. His decision would be made soon. I no longer had strength to endure.

Wanting to get some sleep, but only able to put my head on Tony's bed and stare at him, I heard somebody opening the door. Earlier in the day I informed the doctors and nurses that I do not want anybody in this room who does not absolutely have to be in here. I was trying to protect Tony from any germs that might come in with a guest. Picking my head up and expecting to see Lizzy or one of the staff, I was surprised to see that it was Felicia! Felicia was the first person outside our immediate family who earned our trust to watch Tony when he was only three months old. I hold this woman close to my heart and I admire her strength. Not wanting to be rude, I had to ask her, "How did you get in here?"

Telling her of the rules I set with the staff, she told me, "Look out there." There was nobody at the nurses' station or even outside our door. There is always a nurse outside our door, but not this time. There was no one to get in her way. Felicia was meant to come in this room, at this moment, to give me a message.

As I told her of the happening of the past few hours, she listened intently.

She had a look on her face I would expect to see if I were to meet one of God's angels, a look of compassion, understanding and a heartfelt. "I'm here with you and I'm going nowhere until you fully understand what I have to say. Hugh," she said, "Tony is going to be alright." She continued, "You have to know this, you have to believe this, you need to pray for this and then expect it!" She said this again as to pound it into me. "Tony is going to be alright!" Felicia took both of my hands and said, "Let's pray for this." After our prayer, Felicia gave me a warm smile and hug. Looking out the doors as she was leaving, the nurse's area was back to its normal buzz.

As Felicia left, Lizzy entered the room and sat in the chair next to Tony. I sat down next to her in the big blue chair and started to daydream. Thoughts of Tony getting better raced through my mind. It was kind of like daydreaming about

A Line That Was Drawn

winning the lottery, it sure would be nice to do away with all the bills, for the rest of our lives. But in the back of my mind I didn't get my hopes up too much, the odds of winning are pretty slim. Tony's as well. I'm tired, and I know I should be expecting a full recovery after our prayer, but I wasn't, I couldn't. I was nothing more than a shell of a man. My soul, body and mind were exhausted. I had no more prayers, no more tears and no one else I needed to talk to. Everything that could be done for Tony had been done. Lizzy, Zak, and Mantha were as good as could be expected. I had nothing left. God's decision will be made soon. While staring at Tony, I finally slept.

Chapter Thirteen

I was awakened by the x-ray tech fumbling to get the machine prepped for Tony. When I looked over at Lizzy, she smiled and immediately pointed at the monitor displaying Tony's stats. His blood oxygen level was at 80%! By the time the sun rose it was in the mid 90's!

We've been in this same position once before, although uplifting, we wanted to take this one step at a time. Yes, Tony is making his first bit of progress in over a week, but the doctor will be in soon and will either support our growing excitement or rearrange some of the wires or tubes and we'll be back to square one again.

Trying to be patient, we waited what seemed like days for the doctor's hypothesis. We weren't going to take the chance of missing out on the doctor's reaction to Tony's position, so breakfast would have to wait.

It was about 9:30 a.m. when our Attending made it to our room while doing rounds. Since this is a teaching hospital, he and his students discussed Tony outside the door while we watched but couldn't hear. They were talking for about fifteen minutes when I had to grab the arms of the chair to keep me in place. Some things just can't be rushed, but we've got to know if this is for real or not. If our Attending would just walk through that door he could let me know if I had still not awakened from a dream. Glancing from Tony to his solid stats and then to Lizzy's nervous smile, anxiety was starting to burn a hole in my stomach.

While saying a little prayer and hovering over Tony, our Attending entered the room with a much too long awaited smile. He said, "Well, it looks like we're having a good morning!" His smile never faded while donning his stethoscope to listen to Tony's lungs. "I'm hearing much better air movement in his bad lung." Lizzy and I had a conversation with our eyes. *Could this be for real, is this really happening?* To answer our question the doctor stated, "I think it's time to let Tony's lungs start doing more of the work, I'm going to turn the ECMO down to 80% and his oxygen down to 90%. If Tony tolerates this well, we'll continue decreasing every two hours." Lizzy and I nodded in disbelief. This really is happening! As the doctor left, I felt my body turning to Jell-O and sink into the chair.

Through the rest of the day, machines were being decreased while Tony's stats stayed solid! Seeing this I knew GOD was making His decision. While restraining myself from planning a welcome home party for Tony, I found myself pacing the halls, thanking GOD for his involvement and for catching me while falling off sanity's ledge. Still willing to grasp my hand through all the ridicule and blame amazes me. His unconditional Love was more than what I've ever dreamt it could be. Learning this, I paced the halls in awe.

Through the night and into the next morning, Tony stayed solid with his stats. The ECMO was now at its lowest setting again and his oxygen tanks were set at 30%. The doctor wanted to keep the ECMO on a little longer but hoped to be taking him off the following day.

A Line That Was Drawn

Lizzy and I were totally exhausted and running on fumes. The physical and emotional roller coaster was taking its toll on our bodies. While talking to a friend at work he could hear that we were running on empty. He said, "I need to do something, I'll call you back in a little bit." Larry Brown had called a salesman at Sysco and arranged a hotel room within five minutes of the hospital. This was done with no cost to us. Not wanting to leave Tony but knowing we needed a break to recoup, we graciously accepted the kindness from Larry, Sysco and the hotel. Larry unknowingly strengthened me to the point where I could hold my head up a little higher. This showed me that our support system was vast and strong outside the hospital walls. With this gesture of support I knew the heartache was reaching past my family and onto those searching for anyway to help.

While getting ready for our night away the nurses were able to see our anxiety, they gave us a gentle smile and stated Tony was Critically Stable. They and the doctors agreed that now was a good time for us to refill our tanks and told us that we are in need of a good night's rest. While knowing we could be back within five minutes (three minutes with the optional stoplights) we ventured off the premises for the first time in three weeks.

Enjoying a good night's rest after a hearty delivered meal, I flew out of bed hearing my cell phone ring. It was the hospital calling. It was 2:30 a.m. I knew they wouldn't call unless it was vitally important. I nervously fumbled the phone open. "Yeah, what's going on?" I exclaimed.

The nurse in a much too calm voice said, "The ECMO lines are starting to clog, we are going to do an emergency shutdown of the ECMO by cutting and clamping the hoses." She told me that everything was fine and I didn't need to come up there, they just wanted us to know. While hopping on one leg while putting my jeans on, I said, "OK, I'll be right there!"

When I showed up in Tony's room the hoses had already been severed and clamped. I was told that the surgeons would have to remove the catheters and hoses tomorrow morning. The nurse repeated, "Everything is fine" and the Attending agreed. It took me about an hour of seeing solid stats before I could head back to the hotel.

The next morning the surgeons did as planned, and Tony's lungs were once again successfully working on their own. His oxygen level was in the high 90's. Later that day, the doctor was happy with Tony's kidney function and removed the dialysis machine.

Having a good night's sleep, I looked at Lizzy and said, "Hold your breath for three seconds."

In doing so she asked, "What did I do that for?"

I said, "That will cost us $500. Do it again!" Giving a chuckle we looked at Tony and saw movement, we quickly bolted from the chair next to him. With Lizzy on one side and me on the other Tony was fighting the drugs and trying to open his eyes more than a sliver, for the first time in weeks. Breaking hospital's rules, I pulled down my mask. Waking for the first time, Tony needed to see Mommy and Daddy, not two masked strangers. Then all of a sudden, he successfully won his battle with the drugs and opened his eyes. Trying to restrain our excitement, I whispered, "Hi!"

I heard Lizzy say, "Hey, Buddy!"

With the vent still in his mouth and running into his chest he gifted us a whisper while exhaling, "What's up?" while nodding his head upward. It's a good thing most of my weight was on Tony's bed because I don't think my legs would have supported me. Tony's eyes shut just as fast as they had opened and he went back to sleep. Lizzy and I looked up from Tony to have a silent conversation with our eyes. Our gratitude was too overwhelming to put into words. Our son is coming back to us. Later that day while I was getting Lizzy and I lunch, Tony woke again. This time he said, "Mommy, I'm a football player!"

Lizzy said, "Yes sweetheart, you are, and a strong one at that!"

Chapter Fourteen

After lunch I started to wonder of the price tag associated with a month's stay in the PICU? Seeing that Tony was doing well, I went for a walk outside. I found a bench outside which was close to three people having a conversation. I started to pray about the cost of all of this. While wrenching my hands together I said, "GOD, this bill could be astronomical! How am I ever going to pay a bill like this? Am I really going to have to declare bankruptcy? What am I to do?"

While thinking of selling the house, vehicles, toys and moving back into an apartment, a wave of peace enveloped me with the encouragement of, "Don't worry about the money, you've put me in charge and I am able!"

Feeling weight being lifted from my shoulders the conversation across from me became more audible. It was a worn out looking man in his late twenties telling the couple across from him, "My three-month-old baby is up there in the PICU and I just had to see him. I was able to get a ride up here but in order to keep my job and insurance I've got to get home by tomorrow morning or I'll lose it all. I don't have a car and I'm out of money."

Hearing this I prayed, "OK GOD, you say you're going to take care of our finances?"

I walked over to the man in need, and turning my back so no one could see I gave the man all the cash I had on me, about $27. Walking away I had a challenge for God. "Prove it!"

The next day Lizzy received a call from the parents of Tony's close friend, Cassidy. They said it was Cassidy's idea to have a bake sell to help us with the bills. With Wal-Mart's permission they had that bake sell and were coming up to deliver a check. The next day when Cassidy's family arrived, her parents, David and Jonni, handed us a check for $1,600. I was overwhelmed by the generosity from Cassidy's family and my home town Edmond, OK. After her family had left and I found a place to be alone, I had but one prayer in me. All I could do was look up and say, "Thank you for carrying me when I was not able to walk. You said not to worry about the money, you GOD, are true to your word!"

Arriving back in Tony's room, I was greeted with an excited smile from Lizzy. They reduced the paralytics to half again, and he's starting to move a little! At first it was just an occasional cough, but it wasn't long before his hand was reaching up to grasp the ventilator hose from his mouth. After reapplying the tape to keep the vent in place a couple of times the nurse recommended arm restraints. When she first mentioned this, I imagined Tony lying there and having his arms tied to the bed, how scary would that be for a ten year old waking up in a strange place being tied down while strangers peered and poked at him? Shuddering at the thought, I was happy to see that was not the case at all. It was similar to an arm cast, still able to move his arms up and down, just not able to bend them.

A Line That Was Drawn

Still being on 50% paralytics and the major amounts of methadone and valium, Tony's movements were sluggish. The methadone and valium were to wean him off the drugs used for the coma that was needed throughout. We were later told that if we were to take the dose of valium that Tony was on, it would stop our heart. To us, that put things into perspective as to how Tony might be feeling when he fully woke.

It wasn't long before the doctor came in and said, "I think Tony will do fine without the ventilator."

Looking at Lizzy and seeing the excitement, I walked over to Tony's bedside and grabbed the vent tube protruding from Tony's mouth. The whole room erupted! "Hold on! Wait!" the doctor and Lizzy yelled. "I didn't mean this very second," the doctor exclaimed.

I turned and smiled at Lizzy and the doctor. "I know, I just wanted to see if I could get a rise out of you all." After seeing that I may get slapped by two women at once, I found a chair to start my time-out session.

Growling, the doctor left to acquire an excavation kit. Seeing Lizzy shaking her head and rolling her eyes at me, I knew my time-out session wasn't over just because the doctor left. But now the doctor reentered the room, I got up. "Sit down, Hugh, we've got this," the doctor said. OK, still not over yet, I guess. Smiles in that room were long overdue, and were becoming easier to find.

The excavation went much faster and easier than I thought. They simply deflated the air bubble holding the tube inside Tony's chest and took my job of yanking the thing out. Okay, maybe it was a little more graceful than that, but you get the picture.

The vent was replaced with what we started on, the bi- pap breathing machine which only lasted a day. We then went back to a simple hose running under Tony's nose which supplied oxygen. It wasn't long before it turned into a wrestling match. Tony was waking more often and each time he woke he struggled to get out of bed. Still fighting the drugs, wires monitoring his stats and the painful catheter, it was surprising to see the fight he put up.

Thankfully help arrived. The physical therapist showed up and said, "Let's try and get out of bed, Tony."

Due to lying in bed for three weeks and being deconditioned, Tony needed a lot of help. The PT lady quickly assumed her role as a trainer and was going to help Tony out of bed for the first time. I looked at her and said, "Excuse me, but I've got this one."

She smiled and politely stepped aside while I told Tony to put his arms around my neck and we would stand together. Standing for about ten seconds is all his legs could take. While stating to me, "Dad, I'm feeling dizzy," he sat back down. I asked him how he was feeling; he looked at me, spun his eyes and head in circles and said, "That's exactly how I feel, Dad."

With Tony's continued progress, it was overdue to spread our attention to Samantha and Zak. They had been loved and very well taken care of by my brother and sister's families. My brother John and my sister in-law, Teresa, would watch the kids at night then take them to daycare and school. My sister, Lorie, and brother-in-law, Mike would pick them up from daycare to spend the evening with them and finish homework before taking them to my brother's house so the cycle could be repeated. They did this for three weeks. Every time we would try to thank them the interruption was always the same. "This is what family is for, Hugh."

Lizzy and I decided we would start taking turns at the hospital while the other would care for Mantha and Zak. They were in need of Mommy's TLC and my roughhousing.

This lasted for a week and a half. On the tenth day, about the time Lizzy was supposed to show to switch roles, I received a phone call from her. She said, "Samantha is sick, I'm scared it may be the flu! I'm taking her to the doctor this afternoon."

Nervously, I said, "OK, call me after the appointment."

Later that afternoon Lizzy called back. Samantha tested positive for Influenza A. This was also known as the swine flu, or H1N1. Knowing I wasn't about to leave Tony alone but wishing I could be with Samantha, I sighed. *Wow, how much can we take? Oh dear GOD, not again!* Being the strong woman Lizzy is, she stepped up and told me what we were going to do, "I'll stay home with Mantha and keep you updated, you've got Tony."

Hanging up the phone and looking at Tony I prayed, "GOD, I really don't think we can handle going through this again."

With Lizzy staying at home to care for the kids I was in the hospital to care for Tony full-time. A bright side to this was while being at Tony's side at night, I didn't have the nightmares I was having while being at home, away from him not able to wake and see his stats.

While staying at the hospital, I started to realize what family and friends were going through. Trying to patiently wait for that much needed phone call affirming that everything was okay in order to proceed with the day was not easy. Not knowing what was going on is sometimes worse than knowing.

Within three days of Samantha getting sick, to our relief, her symptoms subsided. So to not bring any germs to Tony's room, Lizzy and I decided we'd stay dedicated to the jobs we were filling.

Tony slowly progressed to walking to the bathroom with my help. After a couple of times he looked at me and said," Dad, I can walk by myself. You don't need to hold on to me anymore."

I said, "I know you can, son, I'm just holding on for me."

Soon after Tony was released from the PICU; but there were no available beds on the floor, So we continued our days of playing cards, watching movies and joking around in the PICU.

Our Attending approached us and mentioned a pediatric Physical Therapy hospital called The Children's Center. Seeing our nightmare starting its end, I happily accepted our invitation after reviewing the hospital online and from the brochure given to me. Also, a pediatrician from the Children's Center came by to enlighten us on the many amenities of the center. Tony was sold on the idea simply because they had an indoor swimming pool. Little did he know, the pool was not primarily used for fun, but for therapeutic purposes. After the pediatrician was finished talking to us and examining Tony, he agreed, The Children's Center would be a good place for Tony's recovery. Tony needed to regain his strength in order to walk and perform basic personal needs independently.

At first the doctors were saying Tony needed to go by ambulance to The Children's Center. But with a little persistence and them seeing that I was capable, they agreed to allow me to take Tony in my truck. This was the best drive of my life. Looking over and seeing my son master the air guitar, while I used the steering wheel as a drum set again, we rocked our way to The Children's Center. It was like hitting life's rewind button. There were moments I feared that these times would only be revisited in dreams.

We were greeted under the canopy by Tony's new nurse, a reporter and cameraman, which we were growing accustomed to. At the Children's Center, not only did they cater to Tony's every need, but they also know what the parents are going through and catered to me as well - three meals a day, a bed to sleep in next to Tony and any kind of counseling I may need. Whether it was financial, emotional or spiritual, they were prepared to meet my needs as well.

Our days at the Children's Center were anything but ordinary. Other than the staffs' apparel and hospital beds, you couldn't tell this was a hospital; it was more like a vacation home for hurt and sick children. Other than the swimming pool there was the PS3 and Nintendo Wii hooked up to a 60 inch LCD to be played while sitting in the gaming chair. Tony and I also enjoyed playing air hockey, working on the many puzzles or playing one of the games that were available. The physical therapy room was huge; there were bicycles to ride, treadmills, indoor baseball, tetherball, and even badminton. The zip line and climbing wall were Tony's favorites, but the end-all was the music room. There were electric drums and guitars and even an electronic keyboard, all fit for a recording studio. Tony asked daily to enter that area and always pleaded to stay longer. All of these activities were fun, but had a therapeutic twist. They constantly worked with Tony on range of motion, dexterity, stamina and strength by adding weights to either his arms or legs.

When we first arrived at the Children's Center Tony was barely able to walk with assistance, let alone brush his own teeth, feed himself or use the restroom independently. Throughout Tony's life he has strived for independence and again he had found himself at square one. We spent eleven days at the Children's Center, on the twelfth day we were playing catch in our backyard. The Children's Center is a place where Angels are employed.

We spent a total of 45 days surviving this nightmare in hospitals. Tony is doing so much better now. After finally being weaned off the methadone and valium, which took over a month, Tony was able to go back to school. During this time proceeding Tony's reentry to school, Lizzy once again found herself with a full time job she adores, caring for our family. I am impressed daily with Lizzy's ability to endure our family's needs. I've always felt it was my job to hold our family up while Lizzy holds us together. It takes two.

The daycare she worked for agreed with her decision and stated her job was secure and was patiently waiting. Tony had physical therapy 3 times a week and numerous Dr. Appointments to keep.

Thanks to Tony's current teacher Mrs. Pezant, and his first grade teacher, Mrs. Smith, he is not that far behind his classmates. Both of them could be found weekly at the hospitals throughout our stay. They would assure us Tony would be taken care of with his education and would lend an ear of support and understanding. We were visited by many teachers and even the assistant principal while at OU. Tony was enrolled in Home Bound and Mrs. Smith would come to the house and guide Tony in his schoolwork. With the diligence of Mrs. Pezant and Mrs. Smith, Tony now has a "B" average, even after missing a semester.

It took two months to get his blood pressure back to normal levels without the aid of medication. Tony is now active in soccer and Boy Scouts. He is also looking forward to getting back into football this fall. Tony now has his lawn mowing business back up and running strong.

I am truly blessed, I have my boy back!

Chapter Fifteen

Throughout our stay in the hospitals, it's hard to imagine getting through this nightmare without our support group. There were daily calls and text messages saying, "We're praying for you all! Hang in there!"

There was Leslie, a dear friend, bringing food daily and her family taking turns preparing a meal or fitting the bill for take-out, reminding us to eat.

Aunt Mary, who lives in Arizona, was one of Lizzy's calls she could make at anytime, day or night. Not only for an understanding ear but for support, guidance and much needed strength, this was one of Lizzy's main lifelines outside the hospital.

Lizzy's dad coming up from Texas as much as he could to take care of anything that we needed, whether it was a shoulder to lean on, someone to talk to or sit with Tony while Lizzy and I took a break. Lizzy's mom flew in from Denver and watched Samantha and Zak for the first week while using all the sick days and vacation she had in order to help in any way she could. My family, Dad, Mom, Mandy, Tony, Tasha, John, Teresa, Lorie, Mike and Rex were always at the ready whenever needed and all of them sprung into action at the chance to help us out.

My brother-in-law Tony, for whom my son is named after, wrote and sang a song while we were at OU, this song can be found on my website.

My buddy Steve and his Mother Pam, brought toys and games for Samantha and Zak to play with while at OU. Steve would talk to me on the phone at any hour I called. He would attentively listen for hours on end, allowing me to express the pain.

My boss, Brian, and Safety Manager, John, represented Sysco with support and gift certificates. Brian would let me know that my job was the last thing I needed to worry about. My job was secure and patiently waiting for my return. Friends from work offered support, even to the point of wanting to pick up Tony's lawn mowing business so to not lose clients and even mowing my lawn searching for any way to help. They were taking collections at work and would show weekly with the proceeds. These people from work turned a large corporation into an unheard of by me, Family Corporation.

I have a new found respect for the media. Worried they were going to be 'pushy and in our face at all the wrong times', it was just the opposite. They were caring and understanding. At times it seemed they felt they were right there in the nightmare along with us seeing them fighting the tears we had grown accustomed to. Three people from the media stand out from the multitude.

There was Meg Alexander from Channel 4. She was the first on the scene to get our message out on the severity of this H1N1. With her decision to publicize our story, she may have saved lives, and I feel our state owes her a debt of gratitude for her timeliness and professionalism.

A Line That Was Drawn

Linda Mares from Channel 5 was not only compassionate about our story but would also sit and chat with us, speaking with us on unrelated matters. I believe she did this to help and take our minds away from the trauma, in a fashion you only find with close friends.

Looking back, during our darkest hours with Tony, through our conversations off camera she would unknowingly give me a glimpse of what sanity was like. She became someone we could call a friend of the family and will always be welcome in our house.

There was also David Gladstone from CBS National News. He was the producer/cameraman. Seeing him doing the story from behind the camera I could tell it was becoming hard for him, being a dad about the same age as me and having children the same age as ours. There were times when David would drop the national news producer thing and we were able to talk Dad to Dad sharing the heartache. This man understood what I was going through and treated me as a friend, not just as a story. I still keep in touch with David and Linda, hoping that their professionalism will become the model of what the media should be and act like. David, reporter Mark Strausman, Linda Mares and Meg Alexander did their job to get the story, when it was appropriate. And when Lizzy and I needed a little breathing room, the camera would be lowered and the microphone would be turned off until the time was right to continue the interview.

This brings me to a man from work. When this man is not working for Sysco, he can be easily found. Because all of his free time is spent volunteering to help others in need. He devotes all of his spare time to the Christmas Connection. Building or doing whatever is needed to assure people that are less fortunate will have more. This man would mysteriously show when no one else was around. He would come up with weekly donations he had taken up from work, the union hall and church and we would sit and talk of the situation. While talking with this man, I didn't have to be supportive of anybody. These were the brief times I could let my guard down. I would often ask if he would like to see Tony, but his answer was always the same. "Tony is in our prayers, but I'm not here for him, Hugh, I'm here for you." Before he said this, I had no idea how much I needed to hear it.

He was able to see the underlying problems with our situation and he became my personal beacon of strength. Someday, when my kids have grown to the point of freeing up more of my time, I hope to be half of the God-fearing, compassionate, giving man that Arnold is.

With summer being just around the corner, Lizzy and I already know this will be the best year ever. For by the Grace of GOD, we are once again, a healthy party of five.

To quote our most beloved, blessed teacher and savior, Jesus Christ, remember,

"FOR THE KINDOM OF GOD IS AT STAKE!"